WHAT TO EXPECT FROM 0 TO 12 MONTHS

THE COMPLETE GUIDE TO LEARNING WHAT TO EXPECT FROM YOUR BABY'S GROWTH AND DEVELOPMENT DURING THE FIRST 12 MONTHS OF LIFE

Heidi Deis

Table of Contents

INTRODUCTION 8
CHAPTER 1: UNDERSTANDING BABY'S WANTS AND NEEDS 14
What does your baby need? 15
Baby Essentials .... 18 Daily Timetable 30
CHAPTER 2: DEALING WITH COLIC 34
Colic and Your Baby 40
How to Soothe a Crying Baby 51
Keeping Your Sanity 55
CHAPTER 3: SECRET FOR LONGER AND BETTER SLEEP FOR YOUR KID AND WHY IT IS IMPORTANT? 61
Reasons Why Longer and Better Sleep Is Important for Your Baby 62
Steps to Achieve Deeper Baby Sleep in 5 Days 63
Troubleshooting the Troubled Sleeper 74
CHAPTER 4: WHAT TO EXPECT FROM YOUR BABY'S GROWTH AND DEVELOPMENT DURING THE FIRST 12 MONTHS OF LIFE(MONTH BY MONTH 78
DESCRIPTION) 78
Month 1 81
Development 81
Fine Motor Skills 84
Challenges This Month 84
Month 2 86
Development 86

Fine Motor Skills .... 89 Intellectual Skills 89	
Social and Emotional Regulation 91	
Physical Development 94	
Communication Skills 95	
When to Worry? 96	
Challenges This Month 97	
Month 3 98	
Development 98	
Fine Motor Skills 104	
Tips For Introducing Toys And Activities 105	
Challenges This Month 108	
Month 4 110	
Development 110	
Fine Motor Skills 116	
Communication Skills 117	
Feeding 118	
Intellectual Skills 118	
Visual 119	
Sensory 120	
Challenges This Month 120	
Month 5 122	
Development 122	
Fine Motor Skills 127	
Feeding 129	
Visual 130	
Intellectual Skills 131	
Social and Emotional Skills 133	
Sensory Awareness 136	
Communication Skills 137	

WHEN TO WORRY?	140
CHALLENGES THIS MONTH	141
MONTH 6	142
DEVELOPMENT	142
FINE MOTOR SKILLS	146
GROSS MOTOR	147
SOCIAL-EMOTIONAL	148
COMMUNICATION SKILLS	148
TIPS	149
CHALLENGES THIS MONTH	151
MONTH 7	153
DEVELOPMENT	153
FINE MOTOR SKILLS	156
SOCIAL-EMOTIONAL	159
COMMUNICATION SKILLS	159
INTELLECTUAL SKILLS	160
VISUAL	161
FEEDING THE BABY	162
SLEEPING	165
CHALLENGES THIS MONTH	167
MONTH 8	168
DEVELOPMENT	168
FINE MOTOR SKILLS	169
VISUAL	173
SENSORY	174
INTELLECTUAL SKILLS	175
PHYSICAL DEVELOPMENT	177
COMMUNICATION SKILLS	178
SENSORY AWARENESS	180
SOCIAL AND EMOTIONAL REGULATION	182

When to Worry? 184
Challenges This Month .... 186 MONTH 9 186
Development 186
Fine Motor Skills 189
Social-Emotional 190
Communication Skills 192
Intellectual Skills 193
Visual 194
Challenges This Month 194
MONTH 10 197
Development 197
Fine Motor Skills 202
Social-Emotional 203
Communication Skills 204
Intellectual Skills 204
Visual 205
Sensory 206
Challenges This Month 207
MONTH 11 209
Development 209
Fine Motor Skills 213
Social-Emotional .... 214 Communication Skills 215
Visual 217
Sensory 217
Sleeping routine 219
Challenges This Month 220
MONTH 12 221
Development 221

FINE MOTOR SKILLS 227
SOCIAL AND EMOTIONAL DEVELOPMENT .... 228 VISUAL
.... 230
SENSORY .... 230 PHYSICAL
DEVELOPMENT 232
COMMUNICATION SKILLS 236
INTELLECTUAL SKILLS 237
CHALLENGES THIS MONTH 239
WHEN TO WORRY? 240

CHAPTER 5: MONTESSORI BABY FROM 0 TO 12 MONTHS 209

BEFORE THE BIRTH 209
SOUNDS AND SONGS 210
TOYS TO SUCK AND GRAB 211   SIGN LANGUAGE
....
212   YES ENVIRONMENT INSTEAD OF A NO ENVIRONMENT 213
MUSIC ....
214
ACTIVITY: POURING OBJECTS ....
215 COMMUNICATION
.... 216 FIRST BOOKS
....
217
LOOKING IN A MIRROR ....

217

BE A MODEL TO YOUR CHILD 218
YOUR HOUSE IS A MUSEUM 218
MOVEMENT, FROM CRAWLING TO COORDINATION .... 219 LANGUAGE AND FIRST WORDS .... 221 SMALL OBJECTS 221
SOCIAL LIFE 222
EVALUATE WHAT'S WORKING 222

CONCLUSION 224

Introduction

Having a baby in the house can be scary, but it doesn't need to be! Written by a qualified nutritionist and a mother of three, this book will educate you on the milestones you can look forward to month by month, as well as changes you can expect to make to your care routine as your baby grows. It will help you Find out month by month, what to expect from your baby's growth and development during the first 12 months of life, and what steps you can take to ensure a healthy foundation for growth and development. When you read WHAT TO EXPECT FROM 0 TO 12 you will discover:

- How to properly prepare for bringing a new life into your home.

- The best methods and psychological approaches to looking after your baby without having to neglect yourself.

- An in-depth month-by-month rundown of your little ones development and milestones for the first six wonderful months of their life.

Don't wait until it's too late, gain the proper knowledge needed to set your family up for success in welcoming this new teeny-tiny addition to your home."

Within the span of 12 months, your newborn will transform from a tiny creature intensely dependent upon you for survival into an active, expressive child with clear interests and preferences. Just as soon as you notice a new behavior or skill, another has already started to develop.

It's a story worth celebrating every step of the way. By your baby's first birthday, she may be pointing out topics for conversation, waving bye-bye, and speaking a few first words. Her fingers will be adept enough to pick up a small piece of food, and she may even have taken her first steps.

The fact is, parenting can be hard to navigate, and there are definitely some wrong ways to go about it, but it's also the most fun, exciting, rewarding experience you'll ever have, and, despite the constant worry (we can't do anything to make that go away, unfortunately), you should be enjoying the unique opportunity to be the parent of your children.

You will be able to tell what your baby is learning by being aware of her developmental milestones. They do occur at a fairly rapid pace, although always on a baby's own schedule, as well as in a recognizable progression. The leaps and bounds that babies will make in a year are the results of an absolutely incredible amount of brain growth.

In fact, throughout this first year, a baby's brain typically forms more than a million new neural connections every second, and it is also the most flexible and adaptive it will ever be.

Many parents worry about how to properly nurture their baby's potential to the fullest. Rest assured, your baby will be learning an unimaginable amount just by being with you. As you hold her, feed her, talk to her, and play games together, you will be helping her learn all about the world and learning how to communicate with each other. Every time you observe her movements, respond to her vocalizations, and seek to understand her needs, you are learning more about who she is as a person and helping promote her development.

One of the best things that you will learn by reading this guide is how to differentiate truths from myths during your baby's first year. Learning what is true and important will keep you on track and, in turn, make you a better parent. Instead of getting stuck on the whatifs, you will be able to recognize that childhood can be unpredictable. Remember that you and your partner are responsible for making the decisions.

Whether you are spending time with your baby throughout the day, in the morning as you are getting ready to go to work, while grocery shopping, on weekends, or in the car while traveling, your baby is learning and growing so much just by interacting with you. When you want to try a new way to play, this book can be your go-to source. The wide variety of simple activities and games are designed to be as entertaining as they are educational— complementing each month's milestones, highlights, and challenges. Consider trying a few new ones each month, and be prepared to repeat the ones that your baby loves the most. In fact, expect her to insist on that. Repetition makes her feel secure while she naturally practices important skills. As you experiment with different routines, activities, and techniques, you will find your own rhythm.

With a love for your baby, trust in the natural unfolding of human development, and, resources in hand, you will learn to navigate the ups and downs of this first year. There is no one "right" way to be a parent. You will always be the real expert on your own unique, precious baby. Enjoy.

Chapter 1: Understanding Baby's Wants and Needs

The keyword here is need. One secret to raising happy kids is being able to determine needs from wants. You need to make sure that you provide everything she needs and be careful when giving in to her wants.

What does your baby need?

Babies need to have parents who are ready to be by their side whenever necessary.

infantparent co-sleeping has always been a part of human evolution. A study by Konner in 1981 proved that close proximity to her mother significantly increases a baby's chances of survival. It is highly recommended for the mother to put her sleeping baby, especially a young infant, in a safe cot, right beside where her mother sleeps.

- Babies need love. Luckily, their idea of love is much simpler than that of an adult's. Your gentle touch, the soothing sound of your voice, and plenty of cuddles are all they need to feel loved.
- Babies need to feel safe. Feeling safe and secure coincides with feeling loved. If you fulfill their need for love, you also provide them with security.

- Babies need lively interactions. Even if you know they don't really understand adult language yet, you have to talk to them in a way that will foster their verbal development.
- Babies need consistency. To help develop their ability to trust, they need to be exposed to consistent and dependable caregivers.
- Babies need to be healthy. It is hard to keep babies happy if they are constantly sick. Proper medical care should be provided to maintain those rosy cheeks and bright eyes.
- Babies need regular diaper changes. Your baby may not cry even when her diapers need changing but wetness can lead to diaper rash. It is best to check for wetness every two hours.

Most parents find it hard to find the difference between their baby's wants and needs. Loving parents dread the thought of upsetting their babies that they give into every single demand especially when such demands are expressed through sobbing or wailing.

- Babies want you and they want you every second of every day.
- Babies want strange things like sticking their fingers to their mouth or worse, in an electric socket.
- Babies want to be your boss. She may not be Cruella de Vil reincarnate but sometimes it feels like she is because she seems power-hungry. She can and she will use her power to control you.

This way of dealing with babies can be seen in authoritative parents. They guide their babies in the gentlest ways possible but they are firm when the situation calls for it.

Baby Essentials
Clothing

Your baby's skin is going to be very sensitive as a newborn. Try not to opt for any synthetic fabrics. Those that are breathable are typically best, like cotton. Know that your baby won't be able to regulate their body temperature as well as you can. A cool breeze to you will feel a lot colder to them, so make sure that they are dressed weather-appropriate. Bundle up if necessary, and don't forget to layer clothing so that you can remove some; if the temperature warms up suddenly. Baby's grow extremely quickly, so don't get too carried away with the quantity of the clothing that you buy. Some items might only fit your baby for a week or two before you are already moving up a size.

Learning how to properly swaddle your baby is going to come in handy. Swaddling is the action of wrapping your baby up tightly so that they feel secure. Some clothing is actually made for this, allowing you to swaddle without the help of an additional cloth or blanket. Don't forget about bibs and burp cloths. After each feeding, your baby is going to need to burp and possibly spit-up. If you do not have anything to cover your baby's clothing, you can expect to be doing three times as much laundry as usual. Buy a lot of bibs, and make sure you have plenty of burp cloths nearby at all times. These are a few things that your baby will not grow out of quickly.

Diapers

Much like feeding, there is a decision that you will have to make regarding your baby's diapers – disposable or cloth. At the beginning of this section, you can take a comparative look at the pros and cons of each decision:

Disposable

Pros

- Throw them away when they get dirty

- There are more size options

- They tend to be more breathable

Cons

- They are harsh on the environment

- Dyes and gels can cause irritation

- The pull tabs can rip easily

Cloth

Pros

- They are eco-friendly

- They are gentle for sensitive skin

- Waterproof bands can keep leaks in

Cons

- Cleaning them requires more effort

- You will have to do a lot more laundry

- They can be less absorbent

A lot of mothers wonder about the cost of each option, as well. It is no secret that diapers can become pretty expensive! They are essential, and you are going to need a lot of them every single day. Keeping your baby clean and changed frequently is what will prevent rashes from developing. This will also keep them soothed and relaxed. Sitting on a wet or dirty diaper for a long period of time is distressing to a newborn. In general comparison, the typical cost for a family to use disposable diapers for two years is around $2,000-$3,000. For cloth diapers, the cost is around $800-$1,000. Remember, cloth diapers do require the additional step of you cleaning them. If you opt for a cleaning service for cloth diapers, this can cost you an additional amount of money, placing you closer to the price range of using disposable diapers.

Bathing and Skin Care

Until your baby is actively crawling, a daily bath actually isn't necessary. At first, your newborn should only need a bath around 2-3 times per week. Start out by giving your baby a sponge bath until the umbilical cord stump has healed. This happens at around 1-4 weeks after birth. A sponge bath is exactly what it sounds like, and soap isn't even necessarily needed. In a baby bath, take a sponge and gently clean your baby with warm water. After the umbilical cord stump has healed, you can start giving your baby longer baths in the baby tub.

Create a bathing routine. You won't need to bathe your newborn every single day at first. It does help to decide on giving a morning bath or night bath, though. Some babies feel more awake after a bath, ready to play and stay alert. Others become sleepy afterward. See how your baby responds, and this will help you decide when you should be giving them a bath. If you do want a bath to be a precursor to sleep, make sure that you swaddle your baby once they are dry, and keep the room dimly lit.

As they get older, they will likely begin to enjoy bath time more. This becomes a great bonding experience that you can share with your baby. Try to make baths seem fun and **positive. Always guard your baby's face as you** rinse out any shampoo, even if it is safe on the eyes. Getting water poured directly onto the face can be a very jarring experience, so do your best to avoid it. You can begin to incorporate bath toys as your baby gets old enough to enjoy them. You might notice your baby splashing and kicking in the water. This is typically a sign that they are enjoying the bath and having fun in the tub.

Your baby can get pimples, and this is normal. **They can appear on your baby's cheeks, noses, and** foreheads. This tends to happen during the first few months of life, and the bumps will go away on their own. Blotchy skin is something that can also happen to your baby; it will also typically go away on its own. Your baby's skin is adjusting to being outside of the womb, so certain things will irritate it very easily in the beginning.

You might notice that your baby's skin is irritated because they keep scratching themselves. Usually, infant mittens will fix this problem and protect them. If nail trimming is in order, there are special nail clippers that are safe for infants. Their nails will be softer than your own, so be very gentle with them. Clip them when your baby is asleep if you'd like to have the most fuss-free experience. When cutting fingernails, follow the curve of the finger, ensuring that you aren't cutting too short. For toenails, they can be cut straight across.

Feeding

When it comes to feeding the best solution for the mother and for the baby is breastfeeding.

It provides all the ingredients the baby needs. Breastfeeding also protects the baby from some illnesses because it gets protection from its mother's immune system through milk. If you cannot breastfeed there are formulas specially made for babies, so you can choose the one that suits your baby.

Breastfeeding/Nursing

Although breastfeeding/nursing is the best solution for both, the baby and the mother, some mothers give up at the very beginning because it is hard to establish this process. It is important to know that it is painful in the first few days and it takes time to get used to it. You need to be persistent in trying because even your baby may not exactly know what to do.

It is important to eat well while nursing and not drink any alcohol because everything you eat or drink your baby will get through your milk. A good, healthy diet and drinking a lot of water will provide everything your baby needs and it will help you stay fit because nursing will take a lot of energy from your body. Food that is hard to digest should be avoided, especially during the first three months.

The fascinating thing about mother's milk is that it changes during the breastfeeding period. In the first few days, it is thick and yellow, and there are small amounts of it because it is all your baby needs at that moment. As time passes by milk changes and follows your baby's needs in its amount and its nutrients.

Bottle feeding

If you cannot breastfeed your baby, you can choose one of the formulas that are specially designed to provide all necessary ingredients for your baby. You also have to pay attention to the different formulas which are usually labeled with numbers to suit a certain month of your baby. Whether your baby is bottle-fed or breastfed, it is good to hold her up after feeding to burp. This way she/he is going to release the air from her stomach.

After feeding your baby might vomit a small amount of milk. This is normal, especially in the first months. This is often caused by the small size of their stomach. If the amount of vomited milk is huge, or your baby throws up when he/she is older consult your pediatrician.

Starting with food

Baby's digestive system is not ready for food until the age of four to six months. Solid food can be introduced in this period. At first offer your baby only a few drops of fresh apple or carrot juice, only a teaspoon of rice cereal combined with breast milk or formula. It is important for her/him to learn to accept new tastes. When you offer some food to your baby for the first time be sure he/she can hold her head straight up, that she/he can sit, and that she/he can swallow.

Feeding a baby is always messy. You shouldn't feel stressed about it. Always prepare something to wipe the mess in advance. Most babies will want to touch the food. It is good to allow them to do that because it is also the way they are getting used to it.

Daily Timetable

By now, your baby will be completely used to eating solid foods. You will not have to put in as much effort to get them to develop the habit. Here is a daily timetable to follow with your baby:

- 7 am to 8 am: Your baby will be up by this time and you can feed him or her 7 to 8 ounces of milk or formula.

- 8 am to 9 am: Change your baby's clothes so that the baby is in daywear clothing.

- 8.30 am to 9 am: Give your baby finger foods to munch on. Your child can have whatever breakfast you consume on a routine basis including vegetable sticks, fruits, cereals, *etc.*

- 9 am to 10 am: Baby can play with toys or watch cartoons or read a book while you carry out your morning routine. Be sure not to let your baby out of your sight.

- 10 am: Feed your baby 7 ounces of breast milk or formula.

- 12 pm: Set lunch for your baby consisting of light snacks that h or she can munch on. You can give your baby vegetables, fruits, meats or other such filling foods. Do not give your child junk food or processed foods.

- 12.30 to 3 pm: Your baby can play or read or listen to music. Ensure you stay with your baby and play with your child as much as possible.

- 3 pm to 6 pm: Take your baby out for a walk or to play with others. You can also take your baby out while you go shopping. Get your baby to take a nap at about the 4.30 mark and wake your baby up at 6 pm.

- 6 pm to 7 pm: Prepare a bath for the baby by adding great-smelling essential oils suitable for a baby. It will rejuvenate the baby's senses and make the baby happy and energetic.

- 7 pm to 8 pm: Give baby dinner. You can follow the same menu as the child had earlier or prepare something else. Follow it up with 7 to 8 ounces of breast milk or formula.

- 8 pm.: Put your baby in bed. Try not to rock or pat your baby to sleep. Babies find it easy to fall asleep if you read them a story and stay close by the bed with them.

You need not stick with the same routine and may come up with a guide of your own to follow that works for you and your child.

Chapter 2: Dealing With Colic

Your cute little bundle of joy has finally arrived. Looking so sweet and innocent, you just want to cuddle all day and all night long. Suddenly, your baby starts bawling and screaming, and nothing seems to pacify the little angel. You are up all night rocking your baby, singing and doing just about anything you can think of in an attempt to stop your baby from crying. This can be so frustrating, especially to first-time parents. Losing sleep when there is a baby to take care of can easily zap all the energy out of you. Family relationships can become strained because of several episodes of this. Parents can become too overwhelmed, and the frustration can make them feel inadequate.

They may start to question their parenting skills and abilities, and depression may set in.

It can sometimes seem like babies cry most of the time. It is expected of them at this stage in their development, because it is their way of communicating their needs and wants. Babies often cry when they are hungry. It is a basic cue for the parents that it is time to eat. When babies cry, the immediate response is usually to offer food via breastfeeding or formula. If your baby does not seem hungry after all, the crying may indicate something else.

Stomach problems like indigestion are more common causes of crying episodes in infants, because the digestive system of babies is still immature. Peristalsis is not as regular and rhythmic as in older children and adults. As a result, milk and air are not efficiently passing through the digestive tract. The stomach and intestines get bloated, causing pain and discomfort. The type of formula (if bottle-fed) or the habits of the mother (if breastfed) may also cause indigestion. If your baby is breastfed, the mother's diet may cause some gas problems in your baby. Limit caffeine-rich food and beverages to reduce problems like this. Some babies have difficulty digesting formula made from cow's milk, so pediatricians will recommend shifting the formula to a noncow's milk-based, like soya. To decrease stomach discomfort, choose milk that is easily digested. Poor latch-on may cause babies to swallow a lot of air during feedings. The air will distend the stomach and cause discomfort for your baby (Propping feeding bottles may also cause your baby to swallow air). Ensure proper latch-on when breastfeeding – the mother's nipple should be well inside your baby's mouth. This position will prevent air from being swallowed while your baby is getting its fill. You may need to avoid propping the bottle when giving formula. Holding the bottle during the entire feeding session will undoubtedly help with gas issues. The nipple should always be filled with milk while your baby sucks, to prevent swallowing air.

Pain is obviously also a reason for crying, which can be from external physical factors.

Your baby may be crying because of hair strands or loose clothing thread wrapped around their little fingers or toes. Your baby's clothes may be constricting the extremities or the neck. Insect bites are also notorious for making babies cry. Check your baby's surroundings for mosquitoes. There might be mites or ants hiding under the bedding and linens, so ensure that there aren't any pests around. Pediatricians recommend using white clothes, bedding, and linens, because it makes checking for any foreign material or insects easier. Regularly change linens, and check for any threading material that may have come undone or loose. Buttons and other decorative materials should be regularly checked to ensure they are securely attached. Better yet, choose crib linens and clothes that do not have any material that may come loose. A lot of these observations and suggestions may certainly seem like common sense, but I want to point them out here, because it can become easy to get tunnel vision and only be thinking about how your baby might be sick, when actually there's something small poking them constantly in their crib, which you hadn't thought of, and couldn't gather information about – be thorough!

Crying can be beneficial for babies as they get to expand their lungs fully. Newborn lungs are less elastic than toddlers and have poor surfactant production. Lung exercises can strengthen the lungs and improve lung function. If the crying episodes become frequent, however, it may have negative effects on your baby's health. Babies who frequently cry may have poor growth and feeding patterns. It can contribute to a failure to thrive. Poor feeding patterns and poor weight gain may result from frequent crying episodes. Abdominal pressure increases during crying episodes and long periods of crying can even lead to complications like vomiting and hernia.

Growth hormones are produced at low levels when babies cry all the time. Hence, growth is interrupted. Intellectual and social skills in babies who cry for long and frequent periods also do not reach potential levels. There could be poor intellectual capacity and poor social skills when they grow older. So, you want to investigate excessive crying as soon as possible and figure out the underlying issues with your health professional.

Colic and Your Baby

A baby may cry inconsolably for hours on end, usually in the evenings. If this happens at least 3 times a week at least 3 hours a day, then your baby may have colic. This a common concern among parents of newborns. This condition is also called baby colic or infantile colic. Any baby can get afflicted with this, most often during the first 4 months after birth.

This condition has been medically described as an outburst of fussing, irritability, and/or crying in an otherwise healthy and well-fed baby. It usually happens after feeding in the late afternoon or even in the early evening. Babies at 2 weeks old usually start to manifest signs and symptoms of colic. The condition generally lasts up until 3-4 months of age.

Crying due to colic is different from regular, normal crying episodes. Babies cry throughout the entire day, but each episode lasts for only a few minutes to an hour. Non-colic related crying episodes have tractable reasons. The crying is not due to colic if your baby's crying episodes are erratic and spread throughout the day. Colicky symptoms persisting beyond 4 months might be an indication of an underlying disease or health condition.

Typical observation in a baby having a colic episode is one of loud, continuous crying. It is high-pitched and often intense. Your baby's face becomes red and flushed from crying too much. Their belly may become prominent or distended. Crying can increase your baby's abdominal pressure, causing distention. Your baby will kick, and often clench their hands tightly. The feet are cold to the touch.

The crying episodes are relatively predictable. It occurs pretty much at the same time every day for at least 3 times a week.

There is no specific cause of colic in babies. There are a few risk factors that are linked to increased chances of having colic. Infants have an increased risk of having colic episodes when exposed to smoke while inside the womb or after birth. Others believe that feeding patterns may increase the risk of having colic, though there are no adequate data to support such claim. Girls and boys have equal probabilities of having colic. There is also no significant difference in the risk between breastfed and formula-fed babies.

Colic episodes may also be triggered by the 3 F's (and one M):

Food - Maternal food intake can affect your baby if breastfeeding. Milk and other dairy products consumed by the mother can be passed on to your baby through breast milk.

These can trigger colic episodes in your baby. Nuts and gas-forming foods like cabbage and broccoli have been linked to colic in babies who are being breastfed. Mothers are advised to avoid these. Also, avoid stimulants like coffee and chocolates when breastfeeding.

Feeding - Overfeeding and underfeeding can result in a fussy baby. Be aware of your baby's hunger cues. Avoid overfeeding your baby as it can lead to poor digestion. Feeding too fast can also trigger colic. Check the hole of the nipple when feeding with formula. It may be too large and thus cause your baby to be fed too quickly.

Formula - Milk allergies can trigger colic. Certain proteins in the formula can trigger allergies in babies. Switching to other types of formula can alleviate the symptoms.

Medicine - Medicines taken by the mother can be transferred to breast milk. Consult a doctor for the safety of medicines during breastfeeding.

The general mood of the household can affect your baby. Anxiety, fear and excessive anger can be felt by your baby, and worsen colic episodes. Air is swallowed when your baby cries. The more your baby cries, the more air is swallowed, and the more the stomach gets distended. This will cause pain to your baby, resulting in even more crying, which results in a worsening cycle. Thus, parents should try to relieve colic as soon as it starts.

How To Deal With Colic

Colic has no known definite cause; hence, there is no definite cure. However, parents have a variety of options to choose from to try pacifying babies during episodes. It is a trialand-error process to see which option would work with your baby. Note that some of these may or may not work, and some may work only for some time. A few tips to console a colicky baby include:

Assess for hunger: If your baby cries after adequate feeding do not offer more milk. It can do more harm than good. Remember that overfeeding would only worsen the colic. Follow your baby's regular feeding patterns. If breastfeeding, give your baby more of the hindmilk. This is the milk taken from the breast at the end of emptying, which is richer in fat and other nutrients and is deemed as more satisfying for your baby.

Try changing the formula in formula-fed babies. The colic may be triggered by milk allergies or difficulty digesting the formula. Opt for a formula that contains whey hydrolysate or one that has a low-allergy formula. Also try switching from cow's milk to soy milk or viceversa.

Avoid giving sugary drinks like undiluted juices. This can contribute to gas in the intestines. Your baby's digestive system may not be able to tolerate such beverages. It is best to give them plain water.

For breastfeeding mothers, avoid caffeine and milk products. Gas-producing foods like beans, broccoli, onions, and cabbages are to be avoided, as well. It could be transferred into the breast milk, causing discomfort to your baby.

It prevents your baby from getting awakened from his own startle reflex. Sleep is better and longer when swaddled. It has also been recommended as a calming method for babies who are colicky. Swaddling mimics the tight and warm environment of the uterus and this familiar environment can help calm and soothe your baby. Be sure not to constrict your baby when swaddling as it may worsen the crying. Ensure that your baby is still able to breathe efficiently even with the swaddle. Thin, lightweight blankets are best to use when swaddling a baby. It prevents stifling your baby and reduces the chances of overheating. Babies have poor thermoregulatory mechanisms and are prone to overheating. To swaddle your baby, spread out a blanket in a diamond figure on a flat surface.

Your baby can be carried in a front-pouch style. Your baby is held upright with the legs drawn up. This position helps move the gas out of the body. Carry your baby and move around the room. The motion may help soothe your baby.

Rhythmic movements may help calm the body. Some suggest placing your baby in a car or having infant seats that mimic car movements. Holding and rocking your baby gently can also help relax and decrease crying.

Babies who are held for long periods of time are less likely to have colic. Hold them even during the day. Parents need not fear spoiling their baby this way. Some "experts" warn against too much holding and cuddling babies, though there is more research that supports holding and cuddling. It boosts your baby's immune system and aids in better emotional health development. The warmth of the parent's body can be soothing. It also promotes good parent-child bonding.

Steady and rhythmic sounds are also found to help calm down babies. As previously mentioned, CDs of ocean waves and gentle rain can be played for your baby.

Medications can sometimes be given to relieve colic. Note that medicines should only be given if prescribed by a doctor. Simethicone is usually given to relieve colic from intestinal gas. It is not absorbed by your baby's body, hence making it safe to use without a prescription. There are debates about giving medications to colic in babies. There is no definite drug that can cure colic. The dilemma is that some safe drugs are not that effective. Drugs that do relieve colic effectively are not safe to use for babies. Medicines should be given with great caution.

Check your baby regularly, especially during the crying episodes. Assess your baby for developing fever and difficulty breathing, as these may indicate a developing condition.

How to Soothe a Crying Baby

During this stage, your baby reacts positively to familiar scents and sounds. Holding and cuddling your baby should be your first and foremost actions. The warmth of your body, as well as your familiar smell, will provide comfort for your fussy baby. Most babies quiet down when kept in a constant rocking motion. Gently rock your baby, either in your arms or an infant swing. Sing softly to your baby – a soothing voice can help quiet down your baby.
Steady background noise can also work. Making a "shhh" sound lessens your baby's crying as well, because it can mimic the sounds he or she heard for months in utero. There are some who recommend turning on a fan, dryer, or washing machine for similar reasons. CDs with environmental sounds like gentle rain, waterfalls, or ocean waves may also help quiet down your baby.

Oral stimulation is a source of gratification in the infant stage. Sucking is a good activity to give a baby who is fussy. Offer feedings for your baby, either through breastfeeding or formula feeding. Take note, however, not to underfeed or overfeed your baby. Either way, it will only worsen your baby's crying episode. If your baby is fussy despite adequate feedings, offer a pacifier. It is alright to give pacifiers even if your baby is breastfed. Sucking will stimulate the mouth. It also provides a distraction for your baby.

Tactile stimulation may relax your baby and help lessen the crying. Giving warm baths (if possible) or soft massages are ideal to provide relaxation. Another way is to swaddle your baby. This gives warmth and a sense of safety and comfort. Carefully wrap your baby snugly with swaddling clothes or blankets. Wrap your baby's arms and legs with the edges of a blanket and then envelop your baby in the entire blanket. Afterward, cuddle your baby and gently rock him or her. When your arms grow tired, you may place your baby in an infant swing or infant sling.

Place your baby down on the bed or crib if your baby does not stop crying, and take a break. It is very important to take some time off. When a parent is anxious and frustrated, your baby will cry even more. Taking care of a baby can take all of your energy. Parents can easily become exhausted when dealing with a baby who cries frequently. Anxiety, tension, and fear can be overwhelming. If not addressed, you run the risk of losing your temper and could even act in an abusive manner if not kept in check.

Babies who get shaken are likely to experience the shaken baby syndrome. This is a group of injuries caused by intentionally shaking your baby. Due to frustration, anxiety, and stress, parents may hurt their baby this way. Persistent crying can also affect family relationships. It can put a strain on marriages because of the stress and frustration. Marital discord, blaming each other and arguments between parents can easily happen when tension is high. Breastfeeding may be terminated earlier as the mother starts to feel inadequate in the care of babies. The incidence of maternal smoking is increased. Postpartum depression may set in. There is the potential loss of emotional bonding between the mother and your baby. The overall growth and development of your baby becomes severely affected. It may even transcend into the later adult years of the child. Frustration and mental exhaustion are no laughing matter – take a break when you need to.

Keeping Your Sanity

Colic episodes can be very exhausting and frustrating. It is especially so for first-time parents. Anxiety increases as efforts to console your baby become futile. This anxiety is transferred to your baby, making him or her crankier, and the cycle goes on until it escalates. Parents may even resort to hitting or shaking their babies. The shaken baby syndrome is a big risk in babies who frequently cry. Here are some tips for parents to keep calm in the midst of frustrating, energysapping colic or crying episode:

Breathe - Breathing exercises can calm the mind and body. It promotes good oxygenation, keeping the cells healthy. The brain cells function better with a good oxygen supply. Also, breathing in and prolonged exhaling helps release tension. Take great care that your anxiety will not be transferred to your baby and thus worsen the crying episode.

Sing - Singing softly helps to soothe your baby. The soft, rhythmic sound of your voice calms and relaxes. Singing also gives you something to do and think about while holding and rocking your baby. It helps to keep the mind off the frustration of quieting your baby down.

Take a break - If all efforts seem futile in calming a crying baby, put your baby gently down on the bed or crib. The physical strain of holding your baby adds to the mental and emotional strain of dealing with crying. Have someone to take over in pacifying the child. It will be almost useless to try to quiet the baby when you are already tired and frustrated at the same time. For colic, the episodes are somewhat predictable. Talk to someone and schedule to have them come over to help care for your baby when the crying starts.

Regularly de-stress - It is helpful for parents to regularly engage in activities outside of childrearing. Sports or other leisurely activities help to calm the mind as well as to release tension. Child-rearing is a stressful endeavor no matter how loving you may want to be. It is a physically, emotionally, and mentally challenging experience. Find time to relax. A few hours away from your dear little angel will benefit you both in the long run. It is also helpful to spend time with your partner as a couple. Go on date nights, watch movies, or have dinner together. Having a baby can take the intimacy and attention away from each other, but your relationship with your partner need not suffer because you now have a baby.

Happy parents are better at taking care of children than unhappy ones. It also strengthens the bond between you, making you a better team in taking care of your precious little one. Take this time to give support and encouragement to each other.
Compliment on each other's parenting skills.
You are both in this together.

Have a support system - Parents need someone they can talk to for parenting advice or just to vent out their frustrations. Taking care of a baby puts more pressure on emotions. Mothers are especially in need of social support during these times, as there is a high risk for postpartum depression. Have someone regularly check on you and your baby, preferably one who can offer some assurances that they are doing well in taking care of their child. Your baby's grandparents are nice to have around once in a while to help with problems in baby care. Parents who are able to vent their feelings, fears, anxieties, and frustrations about taking care of a baby are better able to give good care. Releasing these feelings also releases the tension.

Colic episodes may be frustrating and sometimes feel hopeless, but these do not last for long in the grand scheme of things. Generally, colic episodes start to reduce in frequency by 2 months of age. It gradually stops around 3 ½ months to 4 months of age.
It is self-limiting; it will go away on its own. Usually, no aggressive treatment or medication is needed for colic. Colic is only a phase that most babies go through. All you need to do is to weather out this storm. Arm yourself with

a relaxed but determined mindset to give the best care for your precious little one. After this, you can enjoy having a happy, cooing, bubbly baby, like you have always imagined.

Chapter 3: Secret for Longer and Better Sleep for Your Kid and Why It Is Important?

For infants who are between 3 - 11 months, they require at least 14 - 15 hours of sleep every day. For you to achieve this for your kids there are a series of practices that you should pay attention to and be consistent in sleep Hygiene. Sleep hygiene includes the proper bedtime routine, a clean and safe sleeping place, clean beddings, a room free of noise and distractions, ideal room temperature and dim light. With this in place, it will become easier for your kid to fall asleep and remain asleep for long.

Reasons Why Longer and Better Sleep Is Important for Your Baby

Sleep is very important for babies especially during a young age. The following is the importance of better baby sleep.

Sleep Promotes Growth

Research reveals that growth hormones are secreted during sleep time. This, therefore, increases the need for you to ensure that y our baby is getting enough sleep for them to grow. It is recommended that babies should spend at least 50% of their time sleeping.

Sleep Is Good for The Heart

Sleep protects kids from vascular damage. Children with sleep disorders have been found to have excess brain arousal during sleep, and this can be bad for the heart. The blood
cortisol and glucose are elevated at night, and this has been linked to an increased level of obesity, diabetes and heart disease.

Sleep Increases Attention Span

It has been found out that kids who have less sleep during young age had a tendency of having hyperactivity and impulsive issues when they are 6 years. Kids who are tired and sleepless get distracted easily and are not attentive. To increase the attention span of your kid, it is important to ensure they are getting enough sleep every night.

Steps to Achieve Deeper Baby Sleep in 5 Days

Step 1 – Set the stage

Having a consistent environment will facilitate better sleep for your baby. You should be the one to set that stage before you attempt anything else. According to experts, babies get their best naps and night sleeps in their baby crib. So this means that you've got to start from here.

Make sure that the crib is comfy and clean. The room where you want your baby to sleep should be soundproof. Make sure also that there is no noise so that your baby will sleep better. Consider getting white noise for your baby so that this can diminish other noises that may be present.

Step2 – Start by Planning the Morning First

Remember that your baby needs at least 15 hours of sleep every day. This means that nighttime sleep will not be enough. You have to make sure that you facilitate daytime naps.

The first nap that is very important in the morning nap. This may not necessarily be a long one so don't to worry too much about that because it is just a single sleep cycle.

Afternoon naps are also very important because it helps your kid to be relaxed after they are tired. Day naps should be regulated and you should set up a specific time to facilitate that. This way your kid will fall into the routine of sleeping at that time every day which will help him get better and sound sleep.

Step 3 – Discourage Catnap

Catnapping is common in babies but you should discourage this by making sure that both the morning and afternoon naps are prolonged. This is important and it will help your kid to sleep better and longer during that time.

To ensure that this is effective, do not take them away from their crib. Wait for some minutes and see whether they fall back to sleep again. Leaving them in this sleeping environment will help their brain understand that that time of the day is for sleeping.

Step 4 – Timing is Crucial

Babies of about 4 – 6 months old require 3 naps in a day. One in the morning, afternoon and later before dark. This last nap time usually goes away after some time. It is recommended that the bedtime for babies be around 5 to 7 pm and they should wake up at 6 -7 am. After they wake up, the first nap should start at around 8 – 9 am in the morning. Having this timing is important because once they fall into the system; it will be easier for you to plan your day well.

Step 5 – Give Them Time

After these steps, you can now go ahead and implement the following in five days. With the following daily action plan, you will achieve success in giving your kid a better sleep in 5 days.

Sleep Training Your Infant

Sleep training will work best when you have established a routine with your baby beforehand. An example of a routine may be a bath and a story before bedtime. It may also be a quiet game in the living room before you proceed to the bedroom for a night of rest. Whatever the choice you make, a routine will come in handy when you start implementing your sleep training approach.

After deciding on a bedtime routine, pick a consistent bedtime and stick to it. This means, if the baby has to be in bed by 7.30pm, make sure this is the case every day. Anytime between 7pm and 8pm is a good enough time to set a bedtime. During this period, your little one is ready for bed because they are most likely beginning to feel sleepy without being too tired. Babies who are too tired tend to be cranky and will cry a lot as they fight with sleep, so make sure you choose a reasonable bedtime to go with your routine.

The Cry-It-Out Approach

On the surface, the cry-it-out approach sounds like a torturous way of training your baby to sleep. No parent wants to listen to their baby's heartbreaking cries in the name of sleep training. In fact, many people are strongly opposed to this sleep training approach, with some camps claiming that it causes the baby to feel abandoned which can hinder their development into a well-adjusted child.

In using this approach, you will be allowing your baby to be fussy and shed a few tears, before finally realizing that he can indeed fall asleep on his own without mommy or daddy. And don't worry, as harsh as the method sounds, it is tougher on you than it is on your baby.

Speaking of, it is advisable to try out other methods and turn to cry-it-out as a last resort. There are more gentle sleep training methods available to parents, and these should be explored first before the cry-it-out approach is brought to the table. When you try out these other methods, and they do not work, you will have even more resolve to ensure CIO works as it will be your last ditch effort to bring some sanity to your household's bedtime.

If you want cry-it-out to work for you, it is important that you get started on it while you still have some wits around you. Do not wait until you are at your wits' end to start sleeptraining your little one. If you do this, the whole sleep training will be inspired by frustration and exhaustion. You will be too tired and too fed up to be patient with your baby. You'll likely snap at her, cry along with her and overall feel like a bad parent. You'll also find it nearly impossible to be consistent when you are dealing with exhaustion, and the end result is that you'll send confusing mixed messages to your baby.

The No-Tears Approach

Yes, this is the kind of approach you and your baby need, you tell yourself as you rock your baby to sleep for yet another night. The notears approach is a favorite with many parents because it doesn't involve crying. Nobody likes to put their baby through unnecessary crying and this approach promises that you'll have a happy non-crying baby going to sleep with no fuss every night. But not so fast, what exactly is the no-tears approach?

The no-tears approach, in essence, is a sleeptraining approach that focuses on ensuring that **the baby's comfort and positive** feelings are prioritized over any other need. It aims to create a positive association with bedtime so that the baby can go to sleep without being as terrified as they may potentially be by the cryit-out approach. As such, the no-tears approach often entails doing away with selfsoothing and having the parent soothe the baby to sleep instead. The immediately clear downside of this method is that it does not encourage independence in a child. In fact, it does quite the opposite--it teaches a child to rely on mommy and daddy fully. For very young babies who are less than four months old, the no-tears approach makes perfect sense.

The Fading Approach

The fading approach of sleep training is a combination of the cry-it-out method and the no-tears approach. In the fading approach, a parent gently trains their baby to sleep on their own by gradually lessening their involvement in the sleeping process. You can approach the fading out method in one of two ways. The first way is what is referred to as 'camping out' while the other style is one that utilizes timed check-ins.

For the camping out style, you will need to sit with your baby and comfort them gently while they fall asleep, without getting too involved or attached. For instance, you could simply pat them on their back or whisper soothingly to them until they fall asleep. Gradually minimize your involvement in the sleeping process. After a few days, for example, you might want just to allow your presence to comfort your little one, without touching them. You are essentially fading into the background and allowing your baby to fall asleep on their own.

As for the timed check-ins, you will need to put your baby down to sleep and then check in on them as per timed intervals. This way, you are constantly reassuring your baby without having to be present in the room all the time. The timed check-in style of the fading approach seems suspiciously similar to the cry-it-out method.

Troubleshooting the Troubled Sleeper

If you have sleep problems in your family, most likely you are continually asking yourself this question: **Why is my child not sleeping?** Not hearing any answer to this question from your inner authority is one of the most helpless feelings in the world when you're living in the thickness of sleep deprivation. Assuring yourself that you've tackled common sleep issues prior to implementing sleep personalitybased techniques to help your child learn to sleep will increase your chances of bringing peace and confidence on your journey to HeartCentered Sleep.

The 90-Minute Sleep and Wake Cycle

Adult bodies are biologically wired to transition through five stages of sleep over the course of about 90 minutes. Infants and children, however, can go through that five-stage sleep cycle in as little as thirty to forty-five minutes. Maybe you have been tracking your infant's sleep. That information and insight can finally be put to use. The length of your child's sleep cycle can be determined by noting when they normally wake after falling asleep. If your child commonly rouses or wakes after forty-five minutes, that is considered their sleep cycle length at this period in their development.

Sleep will then often occur in multiples of that number.

In addition to sleep cycles, humans also have waking cycles. Understanding sleeping and waking cycles will help you determine the best schedule for your child. A waking cycle mimics the length of time of a sleep cycle. Therefore, the length of time until your child's body is ideally ready to sleep will be a multiple of their sleep cycle. For instance, if your child's sleep cycle is 45 minutes, then—depending on their age, development, and the total length of their previous sleep cycle—his or her body will be ready to sleep again after either 90, 135, or 180 minutes. If your child is taking shorter naps and has yet to learn to transition through sleep cycles so as to remain asleep, he or she will require more naps over the course of the day. In this case, you can expect shorter times of being awake during that sleep-wake cycle.

Until your child routinely rises at about the same times each day, and takes consistently longer naps, their sleep-wake rhythm and the daily timing for their naps will vary. The length of the wake cycle will, however, remain consistent. As your child develops, the extent of the sleep and wake cycles will naturally lengthen. The principles of sleep-wake timing remain consistent. The reward of understanding your child's wake cycle and ideal times to fall asleep is, again, more ease at nap and bedtime.

Chapter 4: What To Expect From Your Baby's Growth And Development During The First 12 Months Of Life (Month By Month Description)

Development is the term used to describe the adjustments to your toddler's physical growth, as well as her capability to research the collective, emotional, conduct, thinking and communication skills she needs for life. Those regions are related, and each relies upon and impacts the others.

Within the initial five years of lifestyle, your child's brain develops greater and quicker than at another time in his life. Your toddler's early experiences – his relationships and the things he sees, hears, touches, smells and tastes – stimulate his mind, growing thousands and thousands of connections. This is when the rules for getting to know, fitness and behavior throughout existence are laid down.

Youngsters' relationships affect all areas and ranges of their development. This is because of the reality of relationships. In reality, relationships are the most crucial stories in your baby's surroundings due to the fact they educate him the maximum about the world around him. Thru relationships, your toddler learns whether the arena is secure and secure, whether she's cherished, who loves her, what takes place while she cries, laughs or builds up a face, and a lot of additional.

Your infant additionally learns through seeing relationships between other human beings – for example, the way you behave toward your accomplice, and how your companion behaves closer to you. This learning is the premise for the improvement of your child's communication, conduct, social and different competencies.

The subsequent are essential inputs into the improvement of healthful and effective children and adults, however lamentably those issues are frequently now not addressed correctly:

Healthful and properly-nourished kids are much more likely to expand to their complete physical, cognitive and socio-emotional ability than youngsters who are often sick, suffer from nutrition or other deficiencies and are stunted or underweight.

MONTH 1

Development

In the first month, your baby will spend most of its time sleeping. It will probably turn its head to one side while sleeping and will not be able to see or recognize anything that is farther than 20 cm from her when it is awake. It is afraid if there is a loud noise and reacts to light. It will always recognize its mother's voice and will calm down if the mother holds it or talks to them.

During the first month, your baby's hands will be fisted and her legs crossed as if she/he is still in the womb. This will change in a few weeks. Most of the time she/he will spend sleeping and feeding. She/he will recognize your voice and turn his/her head to it. Her vision will be blurred, but she will react to your face if you come close to her.

•**Has strong reflexes:** Your baby can already do so much! You'll notice your baby rooting by turning a cheek when touched, sucking strongly, grasping your finger, startling at loud noises, extending an arm or leg when turning the head to the side, and picking up her feet when held upright over a smooth surface. These instinctual survival reflexes are hardwired into your baby's brain.

•Lifts head for a second while lying on the stomach: Before your baby can learn to sit up or crawl, the neck muscles must be able to support that heavy head. You may notice your baby straining to lift up just a tiny bit. The action may seem small, but it takes enormous effort.

•Keeps hands in tight fists: Because of the grasping reflex, stroking your baby's hand triggers a tight fist. Those little fingers will soon unfold in order to explore, but just like a good swaddle, staying tucked in is the most comfortable position for now.

•Flops head backward if unsupported: The neck muscles are working hard to get stronger, but you need to consistently provide extra support for your baby's head.

- **_Brings hands within range of eyes and mouth:_** Inside the womb, your baby spent most of the time curled up tight with both hands near his face. Look for fist-sucking behavior, which is an indicator that your baby is hungry.

Fine Motor Skills

Your newborn may look relatively helpless at birth, but in fact your baby already has superpowers. The drive to move one's arms and legs in sync in preparation for walking is already part of your baby's secret mission. Expect movements to be quite jerky and unrefined, though they will soon smooth out. The sucking instinct is strong, and those cheek muscles will bulk up, too.

Challenges This Month

•**Feeding:** How much and how often? Watch for hunger cues, including making smacking sounds, sucking on hands, and fussing. When you offer breast milk or formula, your baby can choose to accept or refuse. You'll also notice your baby's head turning away when finished. On average, babies this age need to eat every two to three hours.

Highlights This Month

•**Getting to know each other:** Hold your baby and talk to her. She's learning that she has a parent who cares.

•**Feeding:** You may be breastfeeding. While nursing is natural, that doesn't mean that it's easy, and getting a good latch can be tricky. If you're breastfeeding and have any trouble, ask your baby's doctor or a lactation consultant for help right away.

- **Finding what works:** Practice a variety of techniques—rocking, bouncing, swaying, or mastering the colic hold—for soothing crying.

Do what works for your newborn.

MONTH 2

Development

- **Newborn reflexes begin disappearing:** Your newborn's reflexes are becoming less and less pronounced with each passing week. For some babies, the grasping reflex and Moro reflex (startling) fade.

- **Movements become more purposeful:**

What are limbs for? Your baby is wondering. With this new awareness, you may see a slight reduction in activity. The flailing decreases and stretches become more meaningful.

•Lifts up shoulders while lying on the stomach: It may be a slight movement, but if your baby's shoulders are lifting during tummy time, you'll know that the neck muscles are getting stronger.

•Holds head steady while being held upright: Your baby may be able to hold a steady head position when held upright for a few seconds, and this ability will continue to develop throughout the next several months. Continue to provide physical support until your baby has full head control. Most babies become adept at this skill by five months old.

•Keeps head centered and looks straight up while lying down: You'll likely be noticing the head control developing even when lying down. If you hang a mobile (no strings or ribbons should be longer than seven inches) over the crib, your baby will be delighted at the new ability to look straight up. Remove the mobile when your baby begins to push up on his hands and knees or by five months, whichever comes first.

• **Straightens out legs:** The curled-up legs characteristic of a newborn fades as your baby straightens her legs out and stretches out of the fetal position.

•**Kicks energetically:** Expect a bit of foot action by the end of this month as your baby works to strengthen those leg muscles and develop spatial awareness—the ability to sense where her body is in space. This is setting the stage for rolling over in the next few months.

•**Becomes aware of own hands and brings fingers together:** Discovering the use of one's own hands is cause to celebrate. From here on out, these tiny fingers will begin to unfurl and stretch as the grasping reflex fades. The hands become purposeful tools that help your baby learn about the world. Most babies are able to bring their fingers together by four months.

Fine Motor Skills

It's a time of gentle unfolding and stretching as the newborn reflexes begin to disappear and muscles begin to gain strength. The flailing limbs and tightly curled body of a newborn are a reaction to sensations, driven by the need for closeness and security. Now movement begins to serve a clear purpose. Legs may stretch out and even start to kick. Arms may reach up to bat at objects. Fingers may be discovered with much fascination.

Intellectual Skills

Here's the level of cognitive development you can expect your baby to develop during the first three months.

Respond to Noises and Sounds

The reason babies cry right after they are born is due to the many voices they hear upon entering the world. This confuses them as it had been pretty calm and quiet in the womb. The voices that once seemed quite muffled are now loud, clear, and confusing. If you recall correctly, there must have been a moment when their crying stopped the second they heard their mother's voice. It was because they were able to recognize it. The mother's voice has a soothing effect on the baby as they are familiar with it.

Discover They Have Hands

Their hands will be their first-ever favorite toy. The minute they discover them, they won't be able to get enough of them. Little show-offs that they are, they will move them, bring them together, or just stare at them or put them in their mouths. As they grow more, they will learn about coordination and explore things more by touching them or trying to hold them in between their fingers. They will also learn to open and close them, which means they have developed a strong grip. When handed toys or rattles, they will try to shake them or release them out of interest.

Social and Emotional Regulation

Below are some of the most significant social and emotional regulation developmental milestones observable during the first three months.

Maintain Eye Contact

Although a baby's vision is rather fuzzy during the first few weeks after birth, they do have a keen urge to look at and remember faces. So there will be a lot of eye contact that they will hold with you or others to remember the distinct features of your face. The glances will soon turn into longer and steadier eye contact as their vision becomes clearer.

Smile Back at You

A baby knows how to smile from the minute they are born; however, due to poor facial movements, they are unable to do so repeatedly. At first, their smile is rather reflexive, but they soon learn to do it purposely. As they grow older, their smile soon becomes a reason for happiness and joy. It is an indication that the baby feels comfortable and joyous.

Relax Body When in Familiar Arms

During the first few weeks, babies often tend to stiffen up when held; however, this will change when they begin to see clearly and hear properly. They will sense the familiar touch and instead of tightening up, relax and calm down.

Track Moving Object with Eyes

Babies, by the time they turn three months old, should be able to track and maintain eye contact with any moving object or person. They learn to focus and move their pupils at the same time. They also enjoy watching moving objects during that time as there isn't much else to do other than to just lie on their back all day.

Physical Development

Since physical development is one of the fastest ways to spot development, here's what you can expect to happen during the first three months.

Raise Head and Chest

This is considered remarkable progress if your infant can raise their head and chest when lying on their tummies. They use the elbows to do so, which indicates that their muscles are growing well.

Push Their Legs

When on flat or firm surfaces, your baby should seem committed to pushing down their legs. This is possible when a parent tries to make them stand for a few seconds while supporting them completely. Then lower them a little until their feet touch the surface. They should try to push down and straighten their legs.

Hold Things and Shake Them

As their gross and fine motor skills begin to develop, they will seem excited to hold onto things in their little palms using their fingers.

This is them learning hand-eye coordination. Be it a dangling toy or your finger, they will be eager to battle against it until they have it in their reach. Try to hold a toy near them and encourage them to reach for it by either pushing themselves forward or by rolling over.

Communication Skills

Your child was familiar with speech before they were even born. Every kid has a readiness to learn more, and communication seems like the best source of new information.

Make Cooing Sounds

Other than crying, you can also expect them to make some cooing sounds. They are just trying to imitate your voice, but since they aren't trained that well, an ooh or coo is the only sound that comes out of their system. Cute, right?

When to Worry?

- Doesn't show improvement in head control

- Isn't responsive much to sounds

- Doesn't tilt their head or smile in response

- Has a difficult time following objects with their eyes

- Has poor grasping skills and drops things immediately

- Doesn't play with its hands or move them much. Although you can wait out a few months to give your little one a learning chance, if your instincts are telling you otherwise, it is best to discuss these with the doctor right away.

Challenges This Month

•Routines: Last month may have seemed like a circus at night with the day and night confusion that is so typical of newborns. Focus on getting into a regular routine that feels good to both you and your baby.

•Playtime: Play will still be relatively tame. Stick with simple toys.

Highlights This Month

•**First smile:** Be sure to take photos of those sweet first smiles.

•**First coo:** Your baby is trying to talk to you. As soon as you hear single soft vocal sounds, such as an "ooh" or "aah," mimic them right back.

•**Head control:** Your baby's neck has been getting stronger during these early weeks, leading to more head control.

MONTH 3

Development

Your baby is becoming more and more interesting every day. She turns her head on one side while lying on her back. She begins to look at her hands and opens and firms her fist.

Your baby is very lively during this period. **She/he is interested in people's faces and** begins to make noises when she/he is happy. It is also common that your baby is going to react to feeding and bath time preparations.

Put your baby on her tummy every day for a few minutes in order to strengthen her neck and back muscles. Never leave her alone in this position because she may roll over. Always put her on her back while sleeping to avoid sudden infant death syndrome (SIDS).

Your Baby This Month Your little caterpillar has started to morph into a social butterfly interested in engaging playfully with you. She is likely to greet you with intense gazes, smiles, and vocalizations. She is starting to learn that you can be trusted to address her needs, whether hunger or a diaper change. As **your baby's ability to communicate develops,** the need to use crying to let you know she needs something decreases. Keep being responsive and speaking Parentese.

Playtime is getting a lot more fun and interactive. Most babies are getting a lot better at holding their heads up, and those abdominal and limb muscles are likely being put to good use. Offer toys for tasting and shaking, and hold a toy down low toward her feet for her to kick.

Life may be feeling a little more fun, but remember— **babies don't need to be stimulated** constantly. Simple, isolated experiences are the best. Downtime is important, and your **baby will let you know that it's time for a little** quiet by turning away or closing her eyes.
Follow her lead.

- **Holds head steady for longer periods:** Your baby may be able to hold a steady head position when held or in a supported seated position, and this ability continues to develop throughout the next several months. Make sure to provide physical support until your baby has full head control. Most babies become adept at this skill by five months old.

•***Improved upper body strength:*** Your baby might be becoming adept at raising his head and chest and using his arms to lift up when lying on his stomach. Tummy time becomes more enjoyable for your baby as the neck muscles become strong enough for him to lift his head and look around. Offer plenty of opportunities for practice by giving your baby interesting objects to look at.

•***Stretching legs and kicking more vigorously:*** Expect your baby to express excitement through this urge to stretch and kick. By moving her feet and legs around when lying on her stomach or back, your baby is exploring the way her body moves through space as part of preparing to roll over.

•***More confidence:*** You might be feeling a burst of pride. You and your baby are on the verge of passing from the newborn period into infancy.

•***Time for some toys:*** Since your baby's motor skills are taking a big leap, toys are suddenly a lot more fun. You don't need many, though, just a handful with a range of textures and shapes for your child to explore.

•***Self-entertainment:*** What a delight it is when you realize that your baby is able to entertain herself with a toy for a few minutes.

•***Pushes down with legs and feet:*** When you hold your baby over a firm surface, you may notice that his legs bear weight and bounce. It is too early for babies to stand on their own, but it's not too early to explore the effects of gravity and counter it with stronger legs.

•Opens and closes hands: How nice it is to be able to open one's hands to receive and hold on to an object. Your baby's fingers practice this motion even when there is no toy around: She brings them up to eye level to play with. Most babies can bring their fingers together by four months old.

• Grasping, shaking, and swiping with the hands: Your baby reaches out to interact with objects. Offer a variety of differently shaped and textured objects for him to grasp, shake, and take a swipe at.

Fine Motor Skills

Your baby will be bursting with activity, although most of it is happening in small, concentrated muscle-strengthening exercises, such as batting at objects, grasping and shaking toys, and lifting up during tummy time. This drive to become more physically adept makes playtime more interactive for both of you. You'll want to make plenty of time for your baby to hang out in his favorite movement area on the floor.

Gravity is becoming a point of interest as well. Whether lying down on his back or sitting in your lap, your baby will experiment with foot and leg movements—actions that prepare him to roll over. You'll notice his feet tapping around to find places to push off. If you hold your baby up, he will likely bear some weight. Rolling over may be in the near future if he hasn't managed to flip over already.

Tips For Introducing Toys And Activities

When introducing toys or other hands-on activities to your baby, gauge her reaction. She may bubble with excitement or turn away disinterested. Follow her cues. Some of these tips for trying something new will become more important as your child gets older, but they're good to keep in mind from the early months.

Gain consent first. Instead of directly placing an object into your child's hands, get her attention and ask first. Cradle the object in your palms and hold it out in front of you to be taken or place it nearby. This leaves the choice up to your child. Even though it may seem like this doesn't matter at such a young age, you're modeling respect.

Slow down your movements. Got it? Great. Now slow them down even further. Allow your baby's eyes the time needed to fully appreciate the movements you are making as you demonstrate the properties of the toy or activity.

Respect your child's concentration. No doubt your baby is hungry for the chance to communicate with you, but there is also a time and place for silence. If your baby is beginning to focus on an object, don't feel like you need to say anything. Appreciate this moment of hard work and keep distractions to a minimum. When your baby looks up at you again, you'll know it's time to reengage.

Hang back. Give your baby ample opportunity to explore a new object on her own. This becomes increasingly important as your baby's motor skills develop and she plays more independently. It's okay if there's some frustration as your baby works through something. By not jumping to her rescue and assisting her to the end goal too quickly, you're giving her the chance to learn to persevere and enjoy the satisfaction of her work. If she's genuinely distressed, comfort her and do something else.

Learn step-by-step. As activities become more complex through the months, practice just one small part of an activity at a time and later put the parts together. This way your baby can gain confidence before moving on to the next step. This also works with toys that have multiple parts, such as a set of blocks.
Start with one object at a time, then add more.

Challenges This Month
•***Feeding changes:*** Your baby may suddenly change feeding patterns, which can be surprising, especially for breastfeeding mothers. All of a sudden, your baby may

finish a nursing session in 5 to 10 minutes—he might just be that efficient.

• **Getting your baby to sleep:** Does your baby seem to need you to nod off to sleep for a nap or at bedtime? You may have heard or read advice suggesting that you put your baby to bed while awake, not while being rocked or fed—and that may work for some babies. For others, though, it may have the opposite effect, and you may end up with an unhappy, sleep-deprived baby. There is nothing wrong with soothing your baby to sleep at this stage, and it will not impact her ability to self-soothe when she's a bit older. Just do what feels right and works for your family for now.

• **Dealing with demands:** You know your baby's crying means your attention is needed. It's just that sometimes he has to wait a moment while you do what you need to do. Is that okay? Absolutely! Your needs are important, too. While it is important that you tend to him when you hear distress, a little fussing for a few minutes might be necessary.

You can talk to your baby to tell him to wait just a minute and you'll be right there. And then, when you're ready to pick him up again, make sure to thank him for waiting. If you find yourself getting overly frustrated or angry because your child is crying for a long period of time, put your baby in a safe place, like the crib, and take a break to calm yourself.

MONTH 4

Development

Your baby becomes stronger every day, and her/his senses are developing very fast. During the fourth month of her/his life she/he will be able to see all across the room, she/he will become interested in the texture of objects. She/he will try to put everything that is in her/his hand in her/his mouth.

If your baby hasn't rolled over yet she/he will probably do it now. You can stimulate this by placing her favorite toy on one side and encourage her/him to reach it. This is the time when you can introduce more colorful toys and play some music.

Some babies will start getting their teeth in this period. It can be easily noticedif there are **red patches on your baby's gums or she/he** tries to rub her/his gums all the time. The amount of saliva coming out from her/his mouth will also increase, so she/he will have to wear a bib all the time.

Every week that passes allows you to get to **know your baby's unique qualities better and** better. Daily routines are not just familiar, they are anticipated and comforting. It seems like everywhere you go, even places you personally find lackluster, there is somehow something new and fascinating for your baby to investigate. You might find yourself exploring your home and outdoor environment in an entirely different way. Everything that can be safely sucked on or manipulated by your baby's little fingers is a potential toy.

By now the newborn reflexes that allowed your baby to learn to feed effectively have faded.

He knows how to tell you when it's time to eat and assumes the best position with purposeful determination. You can breathe easily, knowing that he knows what to do and how to ask for it.

Your baby will still cry when overtired or dissatisfied or when your assistance is otherwise needed, but the tears will typically be shorter-lived because he knows by now that you can be trusted to help. Soothing techniques will likely feel more automatic to you as well. In the past three months, you have learned his preferred calming techniques, and it requires less mental energy on your part to offer them.

- **_Pushes up on elbows and hands:_** These mini pushups during tummy time allow your baby to look around to see all of the interesting things in his play space. A few toys, a colorful book, and a baby-safe mirror nearby will be especially enticing. Some may even use their arms to scoot around.

- **_Sits supported:_** There is no need to practice the sitting position or prop up your baby. Instead, you will likely naturally find yourself nestling him comfortably in your lap while you read stories or explore objects together. You will notice more head control in general, and if you give him enough freedom and space to learn how to scrunch, push, and pivot his body around, sometime soon you will find your baby suddenly able to sit up for brief moments, discovering this new ability all on his own.

- **_Rocks and reaches:_** Whether your baby is already rolling over or is not quite there yet, you might be noticing a lot of focused twisting, rocking, and reaching, which strengthens muscles. This concentrated effort is in preparation for bigger, more powerful motor movements such as rolling from back to front, scooting, and eventually crawling.

•**Bounces on feet:** Your baby may enjoy bearing weight on her legs and bouncing. If she grabs your hands and pulls herself up, this is a natural and healthy activity for her to engage in. No need for baby jumpers, exersaucers, walkers, and activity centers. Your baby knows intuitively what exact movements are most helpful.

•**Plays with toes:** Most babies this age will, with quite some delight, discover their toes and even be able to taste them. This allows for a dual sensory input experience that is utterly fascinating, so enjoy this bit of cuteness while it lasts.

•**Meaningful conversations:** The art of conversing with another human being is a mystery to solve. When you speak, if you give your baby a bit of response time, you may find that she enjoys cooing or babbling back to you. Feel free to converse about anything. She won't care what you're talking about, but she will love the conversation.

•**Ready to roll:** Some babies actively twist and turn to try to roll over. When it finally happens, it can be a very exciting and surprising moment for both of you.

•**Laughter:** Your giggling infant appreciates silly voices and animated facial expressions. Be prepared to repeat the games that get the biggest laughs—over and over. Babies love repetition.

Fine Motor Skills

You are likely to see your baby's full torso, including back and abdominal muscles, engaged to the fullest, straining upward and outward. No longer satisfied to simply lie down and be entertained, he has a full agenda: learn to push up, reach and grab items of interest, and roll over.

Some babies will be well into rolling already, but yours may still be working on this milestone or skipping it altogether, and that is perfectly okay. To encourage this skill, notice when he begins to rock back and forth, then hold an interesting object just out of reach on one side. Most babies find rolling from front to back a bit easier. Rolling from a faceup position takes more effort. There are no special exercises you need to do with him. In fact, simply making time and space for freedom of movement with minimum distractions is the best thing you can do.

Communication Skills
Makes sounds like "ooh" and aah", giggles and laughs to playful stimulation

Vocalizes in response to hearing own sounds and when parent repeats baby's sounds Begins turn-taking behaviors in "conversation" (serve and return). When there is a pause, the baby may vocalize to get you to talk more, and repeat this back and forth exchange.

Notices difference by demonstrating different reactions to a happy facial expression and angry or sad facial expression

Begins to notice that tone of voice means different things

Feeding

Breast-fed: On demand or every 2-3 hours until satisfied.

Bottle-fed: 4-6 ounces, 6-7 times/day

Intellectual Skills

Shows interest in faces and surroundings of the environment

Recognizes familiar caregivers and items

Explores and learns about objects primarily with mouth and hand

Hears own sounds and attempts to repeat

Visual

Eyes follow moving things a few feet away when seated with support

Smiles when seeing familiar people

Eyes are working better together (binocular vision) to see farther away—about 3 feet

Visual-Motor

Visually targets objects or toys to grasp

Hits at dangling objects with hands

Looks at the object being manipulated in hands When held in supported sitting, will reach for a toy he sees

Sensory

Enjoys a variety of movements

Not upset by everyday sounds, and sounds become associated with objects

Vision is developing to see up to a few feet

Able to calm with rocking, touching and gentle sounds

Mouths hands and objects

Explores various textures of toys with both hands

Challenges This Month

•***Sleep regressions:*** It's not you or your bedtime routine, it's just your baby. These disruptions in sleep may include going to sleep earlier or later than usual, waking up more often to feed, or fussing for much longer before settling down.

•**_Distraction:_** Like the puppy that sees a squirrel and darts away, your baby's response to sounds and movement is fast and furious. Those more attuned senses mean that she is apt to get distracted during routine activities.

•**_Frustration:_** When babies are trying to perform new physical feats, such as reaching a toy during tummy time or rolling over, you may hear some fussing. Responding to your baby's cries is still important, but a bit of frustration is normal and can help provide the motivation she needs to refine these gross motor skills. Don't jump in too soon to solve the problem.

MONTH 5

Development

In the 5th month the baby can recognize even small objects and track them while moving. She/he starts producing different sounds (growling, gurgling, squeaking, laughing...). You can even make her/him laugh by making funny faces or producing funny sounds.

When your baby is five months old, you can put her in a half-sitting position surrounded by cushions. You can also start playing a hiding game. Put a toy under a blanket and then reveal it so your baby can start learning that things exist even though she/he cannot see them.

 You can also stimulate your baby by putting a toy in front of her while she/he is on her tummy so that she/he tries to reach it. If it is too far, move it closer so that she/he doesn't give up trying.

 Sleeping periods during the night are longer and she/he is more awake during the day.
Colic should not be a problem anymore. She/he still puts everything into her/his mouth.

Your Baby This Month Babies turn on the charm. Those round bellies, beaming smiles, and twinkling eyes quickly win over-exhausted parents and passing strangers alike. Your baby is simply bursting with personality, and the whole world is up for grabs. And grab he will. Everything your baby touches is likely to go right into that drooly mouth to be explored.

The mini pushups your baby has been doing during tummy time are paying off. Your rolypoly baby might be rolling over front to back and back to front, on purpose, to feel that spinning sensation or to reach a toy on the other side of the rug.

Your baby is also getting better at interpreting your moods. When you are happy, his smiling face reflects that joy back. When you feel anxious, he is likely more agitated and may even cry in distress. It's usually easier to interpret his moods as well because he is now better able to express himself through body language and vocalizations.

- **Perfects mini pushups:** During tummy time, you likely see your baby straining to lift up higher using the muscles in the arms, neck, back, and abdomen.

- **Sits tripod style:** If your baby is not yet sitting unsupported, that is perfectly developmentally normal. Instead, you might see her leaning forward to balance with her hands in front in between her legs. Most babies are able to sit upright unassisted by nine months.

- **Rolls over more easily:** Most babies are rolling from front to back, and some are even rolling from back to front. Rolling over front to back often happens within moments, but rolling back to front may take her quite a bit of work. Note: Some babies skip rolling entirely.

- **Works hard to reach toys:** Dangling toys in front of your baby is still enticing, and she is likely to continue the batting practice. If she is sitting in your lap or freely moving about in a play area, you may notice quite a bit of hunting for interesting objects and intentional movements.

•**Grasps with two hands:** The ability to reach for and grasp an object with one hand will be coming for most babies next month. For now, you will likely see your baby reaching for objects and grasping them with a two-handed grip before shaking and releasing them.

•**Music:** In earlier months, music was much more of a passive experience. Now your baby may kick or bounce along actively. She can tell the difference between classical music with an upbeat tune and more somber selections and will respond through body language and expression. But don't feel like you need to stick to the classical genre or variations on "Twinkle, Twinkle Little Star." Play any music that you find enjoyable and expose her to a variety of genres. She is aware and listening purposefully.

- **_Interest in tasting:_** Your baby has likely begun to express an interest in your food. You can nurture her curiosity by offering a clean spoon and cup to explore during your own mealtimes until you are ready to introduce solids.

Fine Motor Skills

Your baby's mobility is increasing significantly. Full head control and stronger forearms mean that sitting without support is in the near future, if it is not happening already. To prepare for this, your baby might do stomach crunches and twist while on her back or perfect mini pushups during tummy time. Left on her own for enough practice time, she will eventually discover that she can push up, or roll and lift, into an unsupported seated position, but this does not usually happen until around seven to eleven months.

The timetable for this natural development is incredibly flexible and requires patience on your part. Some babies master this skill fairly quickly, and others take a long time to nail down the right technique. If your baby enjoys sitting up with you while you are playing together but does not have the strength to sit unassisted, she likely sits in the tripod position, with legs open and hands in between, pushing on the floor for extra support.

Both hands are still working in coordination to grasp objects, which makes sense for picking up and shaking larger objects, such as a textured ball. Many babies will work visibly hard to reach for and obtain a desired toy. You can encourage this natural desire by placing a few colorful objects just out of reach but within clear view. An uncluttered play space with just a few visible toys at one time helps your baby focus and choose a toy to go after with sudden, decisive ambition.

Feeding

Breastfed: Every 3-4 hours until baby is content or satisfied.

Bottle-fed: 6-7 ounces, 4-5 times/day

Moves head towards spoon with mouth open

Baby can hold her head up straight for long periods of time when supported upright

Is able to sit upright in a high chair with support and appropriate safety closures

Shows interest in foods and will lean forward and open mouth for tastes when spoon approaches, and be able to move back or turn head away if disinterested in food

Visual

Turns head while lying on back to look for a dropped object

Eye movements are more disassociated from head movement

Looks from one object to another of 2 objects within view

Stares at a rattle placed in his/her hand

When in a supported sitting position, turns head past midline to watch a large ball slowly rolled by from one side to the other

Looks at a small object (about the size of a raisin) a foot or 2 away and will reach for it Eye rods and cones develop at 5 months allowing baby to begin seeing in color

Intellectual Skills

The cognitive skills improve as the baby grows older. They become more knowledgeable of their surroundings, can remember faces, and reach for toys by dragging their little body sideways.

Discover Fingers and Toes

Now that their body allows them to be more flexible, you can expect them to put their toes and fingers in their mouth or grab their toes with the hands during playtime. This particular gesture is crucial as it helps them learn to turn sideways as well.

Reach Out for Things

Secondly, they try to reach for toys or people near them and aim to touch them by moving their body little by little. This is a great exercise to lead them to the next stage (crawling) as they commence to push their body forward by pushing back on their toes. To encourage movement, place toys of their choice at some distance from them and let them figure out a way to reach them.

Put Things in Their Mouth

As careful as one has to be with what goes into their mouths, you have to understand that the reason they do so is to have a better understanding regarding the shape, texture, and feel of the object. The safest way to avoid getting anything stuck in their mouth is to surround them with things/toys too big for

their mouth to swallow. Also, avoid having any toys with sharp edges around.

Social and Emotional Skills

By the time your baby passes the three-month bracket, they will start to acknowledge your presence. Parents become the people who visit the most frequently, followed by any prior siblings or pets. They view their parents as the provider of their needs, be it for a diaper change, nap, or feed. Since everything in their mind is happening so fast and seems exciting, there is a possibility of them becoming overstimulated. Although it's a good sign, it also means they will become more dependent on you and seek your attention either by crying or acting up more. The crying will mostly end with you trying to calm them down and holding them close. So what you can expect for sure is a lot of cuddles and kisses.

Become Aware of their Surroundings

Previously, your baby didn't care where you took them with you, but they will care now as they begin to make sense of their environment and form associations with it. The baby starts to respond to their surroundings when they turn four or five months old and will eventually give you a hard time when you try to change their association. For instance, if you feed them in a particular chair or place in the

house, they will only feed there and cause trouble when you try to do so in another place.

Enjoy Social Play

By the time they turn 3+ months and begin to see and explore their surroundings, they build familiar connections. So, in a way, you are soon going to become their favorite toy. They will show interest in the things you have in store for them and be eager to get as social as they can in their unique ways. Babies start forming connections and enjoy the company of people they remember. This is the time when you have to encourage play and talk to keep them engaged in play. You will soon notice how their eyes light up and their hands and feet move with excitement as they see you.

Notice Strange Faces

While making sense of familiar faces and sounds around them, babies also learn to recognize an unfamiliar face and voice. They start to mind if they are in someone's arms other than their parents or siblings or people who often visit them. This is another significant milestone as babies learn to form long-lasting memories and be able to distinguish between caregivers and strangers.

Sensory Awareness

Sounds become distinct and familiar, whereas the vision gets clearer during the second phase of the first year. The babies love to explore, which means there will be a lot of head-turning and rolling over on their tummies, so you might have to watch out a little bit to ensure their surroundings are always clear and soft to do that. As for their sensory awareness, you can expect them to do the following.

Sleep More

Previously, they slept for shorter stretches due to their need for food; however, the second term involves longer sleep stretches during the night. Ideally, they will require a good ten to twelve hours of sleep in total. This can be divided into a number of small to big naps during the day and night.

Hold Their Bottle

If your baby is bottle-feeding, you can expect them to pitch in a little by trying to hold the bottle in between their hands. You will notice how they bring their hands closer to their mouth or the bottle to make feeding times less stressful. They may have some problems with coordination at first, but you can help them out a little; however, don't persist if they are not up for it.

Communication Skills

They are making more noises than ever during this phase, and you can't blame them, can you? They have just discovered what they sound like and just want to hear more of the magic they make. They will also show an immense interest in the way you mouth words to them and try to mimic them often.

Conversations, at this point, become their most favorite thing to do, and they can't seem to get enough of it. Encourage this and help them say words by mouthing each syllable slowly so that they can pick it up too.

Squeal or Laugh

You will be hearing some new and creative voices from your baby. Their smiles will turn into squeals of laughter too. This will be the time when your child will make their first giggle or laugh, so be vigilant. Squealing is usually a way of getting your attention.

Babble

Babies have heard you talk, and they want to participate. They will try to talk back to you with whatever sounds come out from their mouth just so that you know that they acknowledge what you've said. You can expect to notice an eagerness to initiate conversations with yourself and others by excitedly moving their hands and feet.

Look When Being Called

Although it is too quick for them to realize what their name is, there is a high chance that they will turn their heads in the direction of where the sound is coming from. They might even respond in the form of a smile or gurgle.

When to Worry?

If they seem reluctant or incompetent to do the following things, it might be best to consult a doctor and talk about any underlying problems causing the delay. But don't be too quick or hard on the kid if they appear incapable at first but seem enthusiastic. Just consult with the doctor and see if there is something you should worry about or not.

- Doesn't reach for things placed near them

- Shows no attachment or affection for its parents or siblings

- Doesn't react to sounds, even loud ones

- Has trouble taking things to the mouth

- Has trouble rolling over on its own, even on its sides

- Muscles seem very tight and rigid

- Body feels floppy without any strength or control

- Doesn't make any noises or squeal

Challenges This Month

•Mouthing everything: More dexterity in the hands means that your baby is better at grabbing and pulling objects into the mouth. She instinctively gnaws on everything her fingers touch. Up your game by doublechecking your babyproofing. Be especially vigilant about potential choking hazards.

•Freedom of movement: Physical freedom in a safe, supervised environment is necessary for the natural development of gross motor skills. Try to use confined areas, such as play yards, sparingly. Your inquisitive baby needs room to roll, scoot, or crawl around.

•Unnecessary equipment: Avoid baby products that encourage you to put your baby in a confined space to practice a specific skill, such as a baby walker, jumper, exersaucer, or sitting positioner. There will be plenty of opportunities when your child has learned to walk to use fun equipment that allows her to explore unhindered, such as riding toys, pull and push toys, and walker wagons (see "Pushing to Walk").

MONTH 6

Development

In this month your baby will be fascinated with touching different textures, so this is the perfect time for stimulating their sense of touch by letting them feel different materials.

She/he will also start paying attention to details and will notice every tiny little thing that is close to her/him.

Your baby is more confident when sitting and her muscles are stronger and stronger every day. It is still important to place her/him on her/his tummy during the day to strengthen neck and back muscles.

During this period your baby will be able to lift her head and her chest when she/he is on her/his tummy. She will also be able to stand on her feet while you are holding her/his hands.

Your baby will react to the environment and will usually be friendly. She/he will feel upset if her/his mother is out of her/his eyesight. If she/he drops a toy she/he will forget about it.

She/he usually uses both her/his hands if she/he wants to pick up an object.

Your baby will babble and sing much more now, and she will show her feelings by different reactions.

When you're about half a year in, the anxieties that came with the previous six months may begin to fade. Your squishy, squirmy baby is not as fragile. Enjoy your baby's relative portability while getting out and about. It will still take time to pack a diaper bag and get her fed and dressed, and yet visiting friends or exploring the neighborhood together will probably feel a lot less stressful. She may be more easily entertained, absorbing all of the sensory experiences offered within a simple outing.

•**Rolls both ways:** Your roly-poly baby might be rolling from front to back and back to front quite often. Some babies use rolling as a method of locomotion to reach the toys they want, and others just enjoy the sensation.

•**Sits with less support:** If your baby has been sitting tripod style (legs open and hands in between, pushing on the floor for extra support), you might notice more stability. Toppling over becomes less and less likely as muscle strength develops.

•**Coordinates upper-body movements:** As the muscles in your baby's arms, wrists, palms, and fingers get stronger and more refined, they work together to allow him to grasp objects with more intention and bring them up to the mouth for continued exploration.

•**Transfers objects:** While most babies continue to grasp objects with both hands, some babies begin transferring them from one hand to the other. This requires the ability to clutch with one hand and release it into the coordinated clutch of another hand—an admirable and extremely useful skill.

Fine Motor Skills

Retains grasp of a rattle when shaking

Reaches and uses a raking type grasp to obtain objects

Holds a small object with palm, fingers and thumb

Releases grasp to drop an object from each hand

Keeps hands open rather than in fists, at least half of the time

Passes objects from hand to hand

Demonstrates a controlled reach—can stop and start reaching movement at different points in the range

Gross Motor

Head is erect and steady when sitting—fully developed head control

"Ring" sits (as pictured) briefly with hands free to manipulate a toy or object Ring sitting with hands free.

Pivots in a circle while lying on tummy

Begins to push up into a crawling position (falling forward initially) and may do some rocking back and forth on hands and knees

Takes full weight on legs in supported standing Will do consecutive rolls across the floor to get to something

Social-Emotional

Enjoys social play and playing with others

Vocalizes pleasure and displeasure with different sounds

Lifts arms toward the parent

Can discriminate strangers

Laughs and smiles

Listens and responds when spoken to Responds to angry voice with a frown

Communication Skills

Turns head to localize sound and voice

Happily experiments making different sounds— grunting or growling, babbling

Has longer duration of sounds

Vocalizes to sound stimulation or speech

Responds to pauses in conversation by taking his turn to "talk" with sounds/babbling

Looks and vocalizes to own name

Vocalizes to get attention and express feelings

Uses consonant sounds in babbling, *e.g.* "da", and "ba", and "ga" sounds

Tips

Your baby is ready for solid food! If you haven't already begun, now is a great time to start.

Your baby can roll over by now, and may even have quite a bit of practice.

Your baby is either sitting up on their own or getting very close to doing so!

Your baby probably enjoys reaching and grabbing at objects and interacts more during play.

Bigger bathtub: If you've been bathing your baby in a baby-size tub and he sits up without support, consider making the transition into an adult-size bathtub. You might get in there, too, especially the first time, to provide reassurance with your presence. Or place the little tub into the big tub to allow your baby to adjust to the new surroundings. Either way, your baby is bound to react to the sensation of being in a larger amount of water. Many babies love it. If yours doesn't, be patient, keep bath times short and offer comfort. Never leave your baby unattended near water.

Bouncy playtime: With solid head control, your little one will feel so much more secure in your arms. Go ahead and indulge in some bouncy games with baby on your knee, or take her on an "airplane" ride around the room. Remember to keep it fairly gentle. Roughandtumble play will need to wait until your baby's muscles are much stronger.

Challenges This Month

•**Drooling:** Where there is teething, there is drool. Sometimes near-constant drool. Sometimes so much drool that the tops of shirts or bibs are soaked every hour. Keep extra on hand for quick changes.

•**Biting:** Your baby has been learning jaw movements in preparation for solid food. One of those skills: biting. If your baby bites you, for example, while he's nursing, respond in a consistent way to discourage the behavior, but don't make too big of a deal out of it, or you risk reinforcing it. Hold him away from you (remove him from the situation) and tell him biting people is not allowed. Give him a teething toy or return to nursing. If he bites again, calmly repeat.

•**Mood swings:** If it seems like one moment your baby is happy and the next she is crying, only to be happy again a minute later, you might be reeling from her mood swings. Expect your baby to have big but short-lived emotional states. It should be fairly easy to redirect attention or calm the current mood with a good cuddle.

MONTH 7

Development

Your baby can sit without support now. Some babies may even start crawling during this period, others will just roll over. Some of them will start crawling backward while some of them will just sit. All of this is normal.

Your baby will probably learn to use her/his thumb and one finger to pick up something. They also love repeating the same things over and over again and trying to copy your behavior.

Easy grins, infectious giggles, and an awareness of the world just out of reach characterize babies in the seventh month. You may find yourself looking at the world differently as you evaluate the potential interest of everything—vibrant flowers, the sounds your car makes, textures of foods—for your curious baby.

•Sits unsupported: By now many babies are sitting up on their own without any additional support for several minutes. You might notice yours looking more relaxed in this position, happily scanning his surroundings. Most will have learned this skill by the time they are eight months old.

•Assumes the crawling position: Your baby may or may not already have been scooting or spinning using those strong arm muscles, but you might notice his back legs taking a more active role in this process. While in a crawling position, many babies this age can now reach out to grab a toy.

Your baby can probably sit up on their own now.

Your baby may be showing signs of crawling. There are many styles of crawling! Some only go backwards, some roll and others scoot.

Teething. Your baby may teeth for a month or more before you even see a tooth emerging from their gums.

Even if your baby doesn't have teeth yet, their gums are good for mashing. Try feeding your baby mashed-up cooked vegetables and fruits.

Fine Motor Skills

Plopping your baby down for a few minutes may feel much easier once he is truly sitting up unsupported. Almost all babies sit up alone for a few minutes by the end of the ninth month, so if your baby is not quite there at this point, he is still well within the normal range. Crawling is also in the near future, although it's still a bit too early for most babies to master it. Once these gross motor skill leaps have been made, there's generally no going back. Most babies absolutely love being upright and perfecting the crawling position with intense focus.

Fine motor skills are also taking a leap. Your busy bee is manipulating toys with more dexterity and purpose than ever before. Most babies grasp with the whole hand, transferring objects from hand to hand as they play. But some babies noticeably start to use a more subtle, defter grasp by the end of this month, starting with raking small objects closer and then attempting to pick them up with more direct finger-and-thumb action.

- ***May show first signs of future pincer grasp:*** Correct and effective use of the thumb and index finger is still elusive. Most babies still use the palmar grasp (whole hand clutching) and raking motions to pick up objects.

- ***Easily transfers objects:*** The ability to transfer an object from one hand to another has big payoffs during playtime. Now when your baby grasps a toy with one hand, it can be transferred to the other hand for continued exploration. This ability is immensely satisfying for her, as the impulse to reach for and obtain objects, bring them to the mouth, and bang them together is very strong.

- ***Easily entertained:*** Nearly anything can become a toy. From the crunchy leaves outside to the stackable cups in your kitchen, as long as the object is safe to mouth, you will find your baby easily engaged.

•**Sitting up:** Stronger back and abdominal muscles make sitting up for longer periods easier. Your baby will enjoy bouncing on your knees, and a bit of hand-holding may be enough support to keep your little one upright.

•**Listens to stories:** It is still a bit early to expect sustained, focused attention, but make no mistake—your baby is actively listening. Keep modeling interest in books, pointing at pictures, and reading out loud. Pretty soon you will find your baby initiating this activity.

Developing a lifelong love of reading can really be this simple.

Social-Emotional

May laugh at peek-a-boo and enjoys getting a reaction

Works for a toy which is out of reach

Likes to explore adult faces and hair
Understands what to do to get your attention

Can discern a voice's emotional state

Communication Skills

Jabbers with vowel sound combinations (*eh, ah, oh*)

Begins to use repeated syllables over and over (6-9 months) such as "bababa, dadada, mamama"

Understands and responds to name

Turns to listen to familiar sounds such as a phone ringing

Shakes head "no"

"Talks" (babbling) to a toy or pet of interest

Looks and vocalizes to own name

Babbles to others and may try to copy your voice tone and patterns

May start to demonstrate understanding of short phrases such as showing excitement to "let's go" or "bath time"

Looks toward family member when named, such as looking toward Daddy when you say "Where's Daddy?"

Intellectual Skills

Takes items out of containers

Understands how objects can be used to get a sound or reaction

Searches briefly for an object when it's taken away

Problem solves by adjusting own position to get a toy out of reach

Finds a partially hidden object

Beginning to learn about heights, distance, and space

Visual

Eyes track an object 180 degrees from side to side while sitting

Eyes follow a falling object to the floor when dropped

Visually targets an object that is out of reach and tries to get it

Demonstrates depth perception

Visual-Motor

Reaches for small objects with just one hand

Starts to coordinate eyes and hands for clapping

Visual information is guiding baby's actions more—how to manipulate an object or how to act on an object to get movement or a sound for example

Will reach for and touch image of self in mirror

Feeding the Baby

Babies aged 7 will gradually reduce the amount of milk they consume per day. This will be a good time to shift them to solid food.

The transition from milk to solid food can be quite difficult, as your baby's body will have to adjust to it. It will therefore be best to take it slowly so that your baby is able to adjust to the new diet.

If you notice any allergic reaction then it is best to discontinue feeding the baby unfamiliar foods.

Fruits are best to start with. Feed your baby mashed bananas and wait for 4 days before feeding the baby another fruit. Start on a Monday morning and wait until Friday to introduce another fruit.

Continue this until your baby is around 10 months old, after which time, you can rest the 4 day rule.

You can check for some basic signs to know whether your baby is ready for solid foods.

Here they are in detail:

- First off, check whether your baby is able to sit by him/herself on the high chair and eat food without your help. This will be indicative of your baby being ready for solid food.

- Next, check if your baby is readily accepting the food being offered to him or her. A baby should open its mouth to accept the food.

- Once baby is ready, give the baby just a small amount of solid food to check whether the baby is comfortable eating what you have given. If the baby hesitates, then make the quantity less.

- Be patient with your baby and ensure that you take it slowly. Doing too much at once can lead to problems and diarrhea.

Once babies have finished eating, they should be given fluids. Do not be in a hurry to put the baby down to sleep after eating. Leave a gap of at least 30 minutes.

At this stage, your baby will not eliminate as much as when he or she was younger. You can reduce the frequency of diaper changes.

Sleeping

Babies aged 7 months will sleep better and follow a predictable pattern. Their naps will not be as erratic as before, thereby helping parents to get some much-needed sleep.

- This stage is characterized by predictable sleeping routines. You will find that your baby is taking predictable naps during the day and sleeping a certain number of hours at night.

This will help you fix your own sleeping schedule.

- At this stage, your baby will not want to be rocked or swaddled. The baby will try to fall asleep by itself and not like being prompted. • Your baby will typically sleep for around 15 hours a day. It will be much less than in the earlier days.

- Babies' bodies will be undergoing several changes at this stage in their life. Right from developing motor skills to enhancing cognition, they will experience a lot of mental and physical changes. This can make them a little restless and cranky at times. Parents are advised to gently handle babies at this age and rock them to sleep if this is found to help.

- Parents need to avoid feeding babies before bedtime as this may interfere with their ability to get off to sleep at this age.

- Now will be a good time to set an appropriate sleeping time for your baby. Your child will get used to this routine and continue with it on an ongoing basis. It will be ideal to put children of this age to bed by 8 as that way, they can fall asleep by 8.30 pm.

Challenges This Month

•***Requires more supervision:*** Your baby's newfound mobility means his caregivers need to be even more vigilant than before. Revisit babyproofing every room of your house. Check for floor-level hazards, including stairway entrances, unsecured furniture, windowcovering cords, electrical cords, and choking hazards. Also secure household chemicals and cleaners, taking particular care with soap pods for the dishwasher or laundry.

•**First foods:** Solid foods may now be on the menu. Talk to your baby's doctor about the right time for your baby to start solids.

•**Distrustful of strangers:** Expect your baby to be a little clingier. When in social situations with people who aren't too familiar, allow plenty of time for him to get to know a new person from the safety of your arms.

MONTH 8

Development

Your baby will start throwing things and enjoy doing this. Some of them will try to pull themselves up into the standing position.
Always stay close.

During this period your baby will probably start crying if she/he sees other baby crying. She/he is starting to feel empathy for others. She/he may also have a favorite toy, so it is good to have the same toy as the spare one in case she/he loses it.

Babies are still extremely dependent, but they are also experimenting with various levels of independence and self-awareness. It is no coincidence that at about the same time your baby becomes more mobile and acquires more communication skills, a new, more socially cautious behavior arises. He is also continuing to take in sensory experiences and is working hard to understand them.

Fine Motor Skills

The wiggles and bounces from the past several months have been building the muscular strength necessary to resist gravity, sit up steadily, and make some big moves toward and away from different areas of a room. Even if babies are not crawling at this point, many are experimenting with a variety of locomotion methods, including scooting, spinning, bottom shuffling, slithering, and rolling around.

Make sure your baby has a large enough space for all of this gross motor work. If you don't see signs of crawling, don't stress. Learning to crawl usually happens within the next few months, and some never crawl at all, settling instead on other effective methods of getting from place A to place B.

Your baby's fine motor skills are continuing to progress at a good clip. The fine motor movements your baby engages in are more purposeful and more effective at picking up, transferring, and replacing small objects.

•***Scoots in all directions:*** Your baby may have found easy mobility even without crawling by scooting around with their arms and legs, backward, forward, and in a spinning motion. Some merely experiment hesitantly while others speed around.

- ***Shuffles:*** Not all babies scoot or crawl. Some master a sweet new move by lifting up and shuffling forward on their bottoms. Others use a tripod move with two arms and one leg pushing off, with the other leg curled under.

- ***Rocks back and forth:*** Rocking back and forth on all fours is a precursor to crawling, which may typically begin anytime between eight and eleven months. This lunging motion helps strengthen muscles needed for crawling.

- ***Picks up small objects with four fingers and thumb:*** The clawlike motion your baby uses to pick up and transfer small objects may be more purposeful and effective now. Rather than using a palm-first grabbing motion, the fingers separate and extend, subtly testing for the firmest hold. Most babies primarily use this grasp through the ninth month.

•**_Peekaboo:_** Your baby is starting to understand the concept of object permanence—that something out of sight can still exist. Peekaboo is the perfect game to reinforce the concept.

•**_Sign language:_** Teaching your baby a few signs can alleviate some of the frustration that comes with the uncomfortable period of highreceptive but low-expressive language skills. Sign language also helps develop gross motor movements, memory, and hand coordination.

Visual

Can see well across a room but still sees things better close up versus further away

Further developing depth perception

Pats, smiles at, and may try to kiss a mirror

Responds to peek-a-boo with enjoyment and repeating

Visual-Motor

Bangs toys and other things together

Visually targets, picks up and feeds self finger foods

Pokes index finger into holes

Eye-hand coordination is further enhanced with crawling on hands and knees

Sensory

Continues to explore textures and shape of toys and objects

Explores texture, smell, and taste of safe finger foods

Develops taste preferences for foods

Able to identify direction of sounds and recognize familiar words

Recognizes familiar textures such as a favorite blanket

Observes environment from a variety of positions—lying on back or tummy, sitting, crawling and standing with assistance, but often prefers being upright

Enjoys a variety of movement in play or when being carried

Intellectual Skills

The baby becomes more responsive to their surroundings and reaches for things now that they can crawl. In cognitive development, we talk about all the new information they are processing in their growing brains, and because interaction with their environment has increased, so does their curiosity. You can expect them to:

Recognize Their Name

A baby's receptive skills are developed during this phase. This means that they understand some of the words and their meanings they frequently hear, such as their name. They start to form an association with the tone, sound, and syllables of the word and recognize it the second it is being called out. This is also true for any siblings in the house or pets.

Have a Growing Attention Span

In babies, this gradually increases as there is always something new for them to tend to. However, in this particular phase, their attention span starts to grow, and they don't get bored easily or move onto the next thing after seconds; instead, their engagement period increases up to three minutes.

Overcome Obstacles

We aren't talking about the big ones, but they will be taking some of the burdens off of you by trying to figure out solutions on their own.

This is the period where they start to develop problem-solving skills and get curious about finding solutions to small problems instead of calling out for you. For example, they will look for their favorite toy themselves from their toy basket or remove a cloth from something you have hidden from them.

Physical Development

Your baby's body is rapidly changing in terms of their height, weight, and circumference, but this isn't the only development they are going through. In fact, let us tell you that they are going to look quite different when they turn nine months old than when they were six months old.

Learn to Crawl

This milestone is one of the most pivotal transitions from rolling over to pushing themselves forward. They finally learn to crawl and use their knees and hand muscles in coordination to move. Some kids, instead of moving forward, move backward, which is also fine since they are at least trying to move. The best way to discourage that is to place their favorite toy or a desirable item in front of them so that they feel motivated to reach for it.

Communication Skills

Babies this age start to understand as well as mimic words containing fewer syllables. They also comprehend the meaning of some words like "yes" and "no." Because they are curious as to what their little mouth can do, they are always trying to repeat the words that have been spoken to them. Check out what else can you expect in terms of their communication skills

Point at Things

They may not have the right words to say what they want, but babies this age surely know how to get their way with the use of hand gestures. They learn to point at things they want and add a few expressions to let others know.

Learn to Say Yes and No

The reason babies learn both or either of the words early on is that their parents use them recurrently with them without even knowing. But it is a good sign that they are trying to be vocal about their likes and dislikes and understand what the words mean. Encourage speech and try to widen your vocabulary so that they may pick up more words early on.

Copy Gestures

Babies might even copy your gestures and expressions if they have seen you doing them. For instance, if they have an elder sibling who often shows anger by throwing things around, they might pick up the habit too if they see it repeatedly. They may also learn to make faces to express different moods and try to copy the way you say things.

Sensory Awareness

Their sensory awareness becomes more comprehensive as they can explore the taste, smell, and touch of different things. Their vision also improves, which makes them better at viewing objects placed afar and maintaining steady eye contact.

Explore Things with Their Mouth

Previously, they were using their hands to touch and explore the texture and feel of various things. But now, they are going to be taking it into their mouths to get a feel of it. Everything placed in their hands will eventually find its way near their mouth, be it a toy, finger, or an edible. It is their way of registering new information in their minds and making better choices.

Sit Independently

Your baby's muscles and limbs have developed enough to carry their weight by the time they hit the seventh-or eighth-month mark. This means that they will stop falling to the side, back, or front when the support is removed.

Their skeletal muscles are firm enough to hold them still in a sitting position. Since they have been lying on their backs for so long, this new transition into the sitting position is going to be very exciting for them.

Increased Hunger

The more energy they use, the hungrier they will be. Since their bodies are developing rapidly, their need for food will also increase, and this is one reason why they will always be putting things into their mouths. And as most babies have their first set of teeth coming out, the munching and chewing also seem quite exciting.

Social and Emotional Regulation

Your baby is gaining rapid interest in you and everyone else. They want to be interactive and learn as much as they can. The following are some of the most prominent developmental milestones they will be reaching during these three months.

Become Friends with Mirror

Your baby will become aware of how mirrors work but may not be able to recognize themselves in it. They will smile looking at it and try to interact with it, thinking it to be another person with the same zest and zeal as them.

Suffer from Separation Anxiety

Your absence will start to bother them now that they know your face. They will cry, cause a scene, or seem tense when they don't see you around. This is what we call separation anxiety. They will begin to cry the second they don't see you in the room; however, this should only be a phase. **Wave "Hi" and "Bye"**

They finally grasp how to express their arrival and departure with perfect coordination between their eyes, speech, and hands. They will be mimicking you by lifting their arms to either greet or bid farewell to you, which will be one of the cutest things they do.

When to Worry?

- Has trouble sitting without support or falls after a few seconds

- Has trouble bearing weight on its feet.

- Holding up the feet when close to the floor so they don't touch it

- Has difficulty standing on its heels and walking like a ballerina on its toes when supported • Drops toys a few seconds later from their palms

- **Doesn't** crawl but rather drags its body forward by lying on its tummy and moving with the help of its arms

- Frequently gags or chokes on milk when breastfed or given a bottle

Challenges This Month

•Babysitters: Leaving your child with a sitter may cause more tension. Allow extra time for introductions, and when you leave, make sure to convey a positive attitude, say a quick goodbye, and depart with confidence (see "Saying ByeBye"). He may cry, but this expression of emotion will likely stop soon after your departure.

•Tasting the world: It's not just toys, it's the whole world your baby will want to lick. Be on the lookout for safety and sanitary issues.

MONTH 9

Development

During this period your baby will be able to sit all by herself for ten to fifteen minutes. She/he rolls over and crawls. She/ he will also try to make steps when she/he is put on her/his feet.

She/he will try to reach objects with one hand and will examine objects by moving them from one hand to another. He/she will yell to attract your attention. It is usual for babies in this period to imitate grownups (coughing for example). She will probably not feel comfortable if she/he sees a stranger.

If you could take a peek inside your baby's brain, you would be shocked at all of the new bits of knowledge swimming about. Those neurons are making rapid-fire connections that will pave the way for new skills. Some are essential for survival, such as learning how to pick up, chew, and swallow solid foods. Others ensure physical independence, such as pulling up to stand. There are also words and gestures to learn and practice that support essential social skills, such as saying the names of loved ones and clapping to express joy. You may even get a hug from your sweetie.

•**_Crawls:_** Those little arms and legs are finding their groove, and this month or the next is when most babies figure out that cross crawling, using the opposite arm and leg at the same time, is an effective method for selftransportation. Some babies never crawl using this method, instead choosing other ways to get around, so don't worry if yours does not master this milestone and instead goes right into standing and walking.

•**_Pulls up to stand:_** Sometime in this month or in the next, most babies learn how to reach up to a low, stable surface and pull up to a stand. While her upper and lower body strength may not be developed enough to hold this position for long, many babies are able to stand up for brief periods.

•**_Bangs objects together with two hands:_** Since your baby's grip is firmer and the two hands are more coordinated, she may be able to reliably bring them together in sync to bang toys or other objects together and repeat this motion.

•**Drops objects on purpose:** Gravity is fascinating, and if your baby is in a high chair, she may intentionally drop food or a spoon and watch its descent. She's learning by experimenting.

Fine Motor Skills

Crawling and pulling to a stand can be a joyful and liberating experience. As cute as it is, the classic baby crawl isn't necessary for every baby. Some babies continue or perfect alternate methods, such as scooting, slithering, or shuffling instead, and then go on to pulling up and standing. These are perfectly normal developmental progressions.

Your baby's personality also influences his level of activity. Some babies are simply more content to sit and hang out, and others are scrambling as quickly as they can to reach a toy on the other side of the room. Remember that your baby may be a few months ahead of these major motor milestones or a few months behind, and that is normal. These timelines are just general guides, so don't let them stress you out if your baby isn't quite there yet.

Social-Emotional

Responds playfully in front of a mirror

Smiles at own mirror image

Shows anxiety over separation from mother

Often can clap hands together

Enjoys interactive games such as "so big" (baby imitates or puts arms up when you say "so big")

Seeks reassurance from caregivers

May attach to a favorite blanket or stuffed animal, using as a "transitional object" for security

Responds to expressions of emotion from other people

Reaches to be picked up and held

Communication Skills

Responds to simple requests when combined with gestures

Begins to use hand movements or gestures to communicate wants and needs—pointing or reaching toward

Responds to own name

Temporarily responds to "no-no" by stopping the action

Shows recognition of commonly used words, and the meaning of some facial expressions and tone of voice

Waves "bye-bye"

Babbles using several consonants

Imitates sounds

Says "mama" and dada" (but may say to others, not just parents)

Intellectual Skills

Works for and problem solves how to get desired objects that are out of reach

Touches toy or adult's hand to restart an activity

Searches briefly for an object when it's taken away

Understands how objects can be used—bang blocks to make noise, shake a rattle, or push buttons on a toy

May look for a remembered toy in remembered location or look for a person hidden behind something

Notices the size of objects, reaching for larger objects with both hands and smaller ones with thumb and fingers

Visual

After seeing an object covered by a cloth, picks up the cloth

Looks at simple pictures when they are named

Depth perception has continued to improve and baby can generally judge distance pretty well

Looks at pages of a book while you read

Shows interest in pictures

Challenges This Month

•***Frustrations:* Wait, the world is not entirely free for me to explore?** This realization may come as a shock to your baby, who was used to having free rein to explore within the natural limits of his motor skills.

•***Staying safe:*** The advances in new motor skills have given your baby the ability to grab faster and pull harder. Your baby has no way to tell what's safe and what's not, so babyproofing becomes even more important.

•***Feeling secure:*** Separation anxiety is still affecting your baby's ability to enjoy her newfound independence. You may find that she is more insistent on staying near you at all times. Many babies develop an attachment to comfort objects as well.

Highlights This Month

•***Self-feeding:*** Whether using the fingers in a clawlike motion or developing a more refined pincer grasp, most babies are intrigued by the idea of self-feeding and will attempt to pick up and move food into their mouths.

•**New motor skills:** Some babies are holding on to a raised surface and pulling up to a stand. Other babies are perfecting the art of crawling over obstacles. Expect new and exciting developments, and understand that before any big burst of development often comes a slight regression or plateau.

•**Encouragement:** Your baby is working hard and looking to you for emotional support and a positive attitude about his hard work. As he accomplishes new things, he's feeling the intrinsic reward and satisfaction from his efforts paying off.

MONTH 10

Development

Your baby's personality is becoming more and more developed. She/he is trying to understand everything you say to her/him and tries to react. Some babies will know to wave goodbye in this period, others will try to speak. The most important thing for you is to encourage her/his development in every way. Try to explain things you do while talking to your baby. This will help her/him acknowledge certain words. Even though she/he won't be able to say the word correctly, this will help her/him recognize it.

Your little one has been growing outside of the womb for about as long as a typical pregnancy. And just look at the vast amount of growth that has happened during that time! You now have an inquisitive and communicative family member with original thoughts, feelings, and ideas to share with the world.

Flexibility and mobility have taken another big leap. Getting around from place to place, manipulating intriguing objects, and even a menu of favorite foods isn't so tough anymore. In fact, it might feel so easy to crawl off to play independently that your baby has, in response, become even more attached to you and aware of your presence. This is a natural instinct for protection. She will be instinctively trying all kinds of new things, and some of those will be a little risky. Keeping a parent close by just makes sense from her perspective. Now is the time to teach her what foods are good to eat, what toys are safe to play with, and how to have a back-and-forth conversation.

- **Switches positions:** From sitting to crawling to pulling up, then back to sitting and craning over sideways, babies are learning to change body positions impulsively with much less effort than before.

- **Pulls to a stand and balances:** By the end of this month, many babies are pulling up to a stand, and some are even able to stand alone unsupported for a few seconds. Cruising is also a possibility either now or in the near future, as your baby is looking for surfaces to hold on to for support in learning to walk.

- **Refines the pincer grip:** Your baby may be making more attempts to use the thumb and index finger in coordination to pick up tiny objects, a skill that eases self-feeding. Most one-year-olds have mastered this skill.

Manipulates objects: Those busy little fingers are working hard to effect change on objects. You might

- notice that your baby is exploring how to open and close, push and pull, twist and turn all kinds of objects. The primary purpose is practicing fine motor skills and exploring the properties, not necessarily using the object for its intended purpose.

- **Learns to let go voluntarily:** Up until around now, your baby's primary motivation when it came to obtaining objects was to clutch and hold it until it fell of its own accord. Last month, you might have noticed him beginning to experiment with dropping items. This month, you might be seeing more muscle control involved as he purposefully lets go of an object and observes the effect.

- **First words:** Some babies are saying a first word or two this month, and that is something that many parents like to record and remember with fondness later on.

- **Copycat games:** Back-and-forth vocalizations and movements are hugely appealing to most babies. Get your silly on, because your baby will enjoy being your mirror and letting you do the imitating, too.

- **Messy play:** Self-feeding alone provides plenty of opportunities for messy play, but your baby also might enjoy feeling the squishy mud outdoors or crawling through a pile of leaves. Whatever you do, don't shy away from sensory experiences because of a possible mess. It's a developmentally appropriate part of your baby's education.

Fine Motor Skills

Keeping up with your baby may feel like trying to chase a rolling ball down a hill. Many babies will not be afraid in the least to aim and lunge for exactly what they want to explore, and once they get there, they may quickly move along to the next enticing thing. Fortunately, the motor skills your baby has been practicing for the last nine months are being put to good use, and your baby is likely practicing switching from one type of movement to the other on a whim.

Entertaining your little ball of energy doesn't need to be difficult. Make sure that you are keeping floor space open for big movements and providing a regular rotation of interesting objects to manipulate. The fine motor skills are continuing to develop just as quickly as the gross motor skills. Babies tend to be especially interested in pinching, pulling, and letting go of objects.

Social-Emotional

Waves "bye-bye" or may blow kisses

Plays pat-a-cake

Gives affection

May continue with signs of separation anxiety

Generally happy when not hungry or tired Reaches arms to be picked up

Imitates other children and mimics simple actions

Develops confidence that he can finger feed himself

Communication Skills

Can understand and follow simple requests such as "wave bye-bye", "clap hands", or "give me the toy"

Baby may point to or reach toward an object that you name

Produces longer strings of jargon in social communication with more intonation

Explores different sounds that he/she can make and imitates sounds

May correctly refer to each parent as "mama or "dada"

Intellectual Skills

Puts objects in and out of containers

Begins to use familiar objects in the correct function (spoon to mouth, comb to hair)— imitates you using common, frequently used objects (toy phone to ear)

Retains 2 objects in hand and reaches for a 3rd

Starting to understand and learn spatial relationships, especially if talked about in play—on/off, up/down, under/over

Visual

Looks closely at tiny objects

Gazes at or in the direction of a named object

Able to better focus on quickly moving objects

Looks at and scans pages of book as you read Visual-

Motor

Removes items from containers, picking things out or dumping them out

Imitates using 2 different objects, such as hitting a cup with a spoon

Slides an object, (like a car) on a surface

Claps hands several times

Pulls on a string to get the attached toy

Releases a block into an adult's held out palm

Sensory

Enjoys a greater variety of tastes

Developing food preferences—may take 10 tries before baby learns to like a new food

Baby is getting around more, and therefore exploring textures through touching a variety of objects and surfaces

Enjoys and explores a wide variety of touch, noises and smells

Usually does not startle to everyday sounds Able to calm with rocking, holding, and to your voice or singing

Increase in smell and taste preference, and intensity of reaction

Continues to investigates shapes, sizes and textures with hands and explores with mouth

Observes environment from a variety of positions and enjoys playful movement in different directions and positions

Challenges This Month

•***Playgroup playtime:*** Taking your baby to a playgroup can be a fun and helpful experience for both of you, but it has some challenges. Babies of this age don't actually play together; they play parallel to each other, and they may be upset when a toy is grabbed away.

•***Bumps and bruises:*** If your baby is pulling up on furniture or crawling fairly quickly, you may see some bruises appear after a tumble.

Common places for bumps and bruises include the forehead, elbows, knees, and shins.

- **New fears:** Aside from the separation anxiety that is so common, your baby may suddenly become fearful of familiar sounds and objects. Common new fears include the vacuum cleaner, the toilet flushing, and barking dogs. For most children, this is temporary. Try to remain calm and comforting, but don't overreact or force your child to have a close encounter with the source of these troubled emotions. These worries typically subside on their own.

MONTH 11

Development

Your baby is active almost every moment of the day she is awake. Sometimes you miss that period from the first weeks when she was mostly sleeping and eating. Now everything seems interesting to her/him and she/he is constantly exploring around the house. You should be really cautious during this period and never leave your baby out of sight.

Your Baby This Month Your baby is probably looking much more like an active, busy toddler than a baby. Your life together is changing every day as you approach the end of the first year.

The world is full of fascinating objects to manipulate, foods to try, and people to meet, even if your little one feels shy around strangers. The close and trusting relationship you have worked to build with him since the moment of birth is a gift for your future together. As he grows into more of an independent being and begins to slowly separate from you psychologically and physically, that secure bond will be even more appreciated.

•***Sits from a standing position:*** Most babies are getting pretty good at standing by this month, and some are even sitting down from standing without losing balance or toppling backward. This new ability bolsters confidence while cruising because your baby knows that any time he feels unstable, sitting down is always an option.

•***Holds your hand to stand:*** If you hold out a hand, your baby may just take it and pull up to a stand. Knowing that you are close by for emotional and physical assistance can make all the difference in his desire to keep practicing pulling up and holding the position.

•***Stands alone for brief periods:*** Some babies are getting so comfortable pulling up and standing that they are successful in letting go for a few seconds. A few even take a few steps before sitting back down.

•***Cruises around the furniture:*** Furniture may have become a gym for gross motor development. Many babies practice cruising from one piece of furniture to the next, pausing to crawl to the next place to pull up.

- ***Dumps and fills containers:*** While fine motor skills are still a big focus for this month, you might notice your baby squealing with glee while dumping out objects onto the floor.

Support this developmental need by providing open containers, such as baskets or bowls, that your baby can fill with interesting objects. He can then dump everything out and start again.

- ***Playing ball:*** Sometime soon, if not already, your baby will be capable of rolling a ball back and forth with you. Sit a few feet away with your legs spread apart and roll the ball to your baby. She may choose to catch and roll the ball back to you or explore its properties on her own. Either decision is fine and will lead to learning opportunities for your little one.

- ***Making choices:*** Your baby is able to show you more clearly which of two items is preferred, so offering her simple choices gently introduces her to a more independent lifestyle.

When offering choices, make sure that both options are safe and acceptable.

•***Receptive language:*** Listening to your adult speech is critical. Using short, clear sentences when communicating with your baby is fine and aids his comprehension, but try not to use much baby talk to change the words and phrases themselves. Your baby is listening very intently for the correct pronunciation to imitate.

Fine Motor Skills

Most babies are pulling up fairly well and practicing some standing and cruising. When your baby starts moving around upright, his gait likely starts with an adorable waddling, back-and-forth rocking motion. This extra momentum is usually needed to propel his body forward effectively. These initial attempts become smoother and smoother with practice.

You may enjoy holding your little one's hand, although at this stage the desire for actual hand-holding will not be mutual. Instead, think of yourself as offering another stable place for support, both moral and physical. Let your baby take the lead here and do all of the balancing work. Resist the urge to offer too much assistance. Keep your arms steady and your grip loose. You want to bolster confidence, but you don't want him to throw caution to the wind. That bit of caution and the knowledge of his current capabilities will come in handy when encountering a flight of stairs.

Social-Emotional
Extends toy to a person but may not release Leaves physical contact with a person momentarily

Enjoys interacting with familiar people in play

Performs for social attention—repeats action/activity that gets a response from others

Imitates facial expressions

May strongly express likes and dislikes, learning to use their emotions to get what they want

May show fear with new situations

Communication Skills

Imitates sounds of words

Imitates consonant-vowel combinations

Performs on verbal cue alone (without gesture or modeling)

Imitates non-speech sounds (click, cough)

Baby is learning that words represent a thing, person or action—looks at familiar objects or persons when named

Stops or pauses activity in response to "no"

Engages in back and forth exchanges

Babbling has sounds and rhythms of speech

Refers to "mama" and "dada" correctly

Imperfectly imitates new movement never performed before

Finds and obtains a completely hidden object, even if he didn't see you hide the object

Takes ring stacks off of a pole

Visual

Finds a small toy after watching you hide it entirely under a cloth

Visually tracks a ball rolling down an incline

Sees well near and far and can focus on objects moving quickly

Can recognize familiar people when looking through a window

Recognizes pictures

Sensory

Continues to develop food preferences—may take 10 tries before baby learns to like a new food

Enjoys touch of favorite blanket, stuffed animal or toy

Starts to investigate objects more through touch than through the mouth

Baby's vestibular system (located in the inner ear), vision, and the ability to process information about body position through muscles and joints, and sense of touch are all coordinating together to help him orient in space, balance, and move efficiently to perform a task at hand.

Enjoys a wide variety of music/sounds, touch and movement play

May turn head away from strong smells

Enjoys exploring messy play especially with food

Sleeping routine

- You can set an appropriate bedtime so that your baby can fall asleep at the same time every day.

- Your baby will not sleep so much during the daytime. He or she will take only a couple of predictable naps.

- Now will be a great time to move your baby to his or her own room or cot. Babies of this age find it easier to transition and prefer to sleep on their own.

- You can prepare a nice room for your baby and ensure the atmosphere is tailored to the child's needs. Right from the lighting to the temperature, ensure that everything is perfect for your baby. Stay with your baby until the baby gets accustomed to being in this room and falls asleep.

Challenges This Month

- **Naps:** Babies who take the typical morning and afternoon naps may soon drop one. The morning nap is typically dropped first, but not always. Some babies will attempt to stop napping altogether because playtime has become such fun. While you can't make a baby fall asleep or stay asleep, the right environment and a consistent routine can be effective encouragement. Even if she stays awake during naptime, having regular quiet time can give her a chance to recharge.

•**Listening:** The world is so captivating that getting your baby's attention might require more effort on your part. To make sure your baby is listening to you, get close, look into her eyes, and maintain eye contact. Speaking in a soft voice up close is also often more effective than yelling from afar.

•**Tipping objects over:** Your home may feel like a disaster zone by the time your baby is done with playtime. For the next year, your little one will find cause and effect absolutely delightful, but you might find it tiresome as you pick up the toys she drops and scatters on purpose. Keep the selection of toys to a manageable level, and use open storage—for example, small baskets or a low shelf that your baby can access. If you keep calmly modeling how to put items back where they belong and make the process simple, your toddler will start to emulate this behavior in the next several months.

MONTH 12

Development

Your baby is not a baby anymore. She/he can do so many things. She/he understands most things you say to her/him. You can even teach her/him to collect toys. She/he will be able to understand the word "no", although she/he will probably ignore it.

She/he will especially be fascinated with colorful books for that age. It is also important to continue encouraging your baby to speak. Always repeat the words, count steps while you are climbing the stairs... Repetition will lead to remembering, no matter how silly it may look for you.

Your baby may enjoy picking up small objects using their thumb, pointer and middle fingers. This is called the "pincer" grasp. Encourage the development of this grasp by providing small cooked vegetables and crackers or cereal to pick up.

Your baby's first tantrums may begin if they haven't already. Your baby's memory is getting stronger and they may remember what you've said "no" to. However, redirection is a great tactic to manage these outbursts. If you say no to a lollipop or grabbing a knife, offer something else to fulfill your baby's needs.

Your little baby will soon be one year old. Whether he's still crawling for a few months or already toddling about, life with your little one will be different next year. The two of you are both well prepared now for all of the changes in development coming your way. Every time you sat down to rock, feed, sing a lullaby, or whisper words of love, you were calming the nervous system, setting the stage for a secure attachment that has a lifetime of emotional benefits. Your baby is now learning to feel like a separate person with original thoughts, physical independence, and more complex goals.

Your baby is taking on more complicated activities, which require more concentration. When he makes what look to you like mistakes, resist any temptation to jump in and show him what you see as the correct or more efficient way to do things. Hold yourself back from helping too soon and too often, and he will learn a lesson much greater than any separate skill: perseverance. Trust in your child, and enter the next year with confidence.

•**Playground adventures:** Your little mountaineer may be excited to climb and explore new heights. Playgrounds can be full of older children who aren't watching out for your baby, so you'll need to supervise extra closely while you enjoy exploring these new challenges together.

- **Affection:** Your baby has more selfawareness and will let you know how appreciated you are in many ways, even if they are still primarily nonverbal. When she gives you brief hugs and wet kisses, reaches up to be in your arms, and cries when you're out of sight, you know that you are well loved.

- **Stoops from a standing position:** By the end of this month, about a quarter of babies will be practicing bending over and standing straight back up again. When a toy is dropped onto the floor, it will be much easier for your baby to bend over to pick it up. You may even see your baby do this over and over again on purpose to practice this skill.

- **Turns pages of a book:** The pincer grasp is being put to very good use when reading a book together. If you lift and hold a page out steady, your baby may be able to pinch the corner and turn it over so that you can read the next one. This is a preliteracy skill.

•***May take first steps:*** No one can tell you exactly when your baby will take those first steps, but when he does, a real toddler isn't too far off. To encourage this milestone, allow lots of time for your baby to practice cruising and balancing while standing still.

• ***Transfers objects:*** Your baby is getting more adept at picking up objects from one spot and transferring them to another spot. At first, your baby will likely be working with only one container, such as taking balls in and out of a basket. When this skill is well developed, your baby will work with two containers at a time, transferring objects back and forth between them. You might even see your baby holding two objects in one hand while working with the other hand.

Fine Motor Skills

Either way, your job is mostly to have patience, giving your baby the time and physical freedom to learn this new, lifechanging skill. If she still isn't walking by about 18 months, bring it up with your baby's doctor. Otherwise, enjoy those cute crawling or shuffling movements while they last and trust that your baby is developing at the perfect pace.

Social and Emotional Development

These months are great for parents because their child finally learns of and acknowledges the special bond that they have with you, their siblings, and relatives. Some of the most prominent characteristics to look for during this stage include the following.

Resist Change or Have Specific Demands

As they are moving to become more independent, they will have some very specific demands they want catered to. For example, they might insist on wearing another shirt than the one you laid out, resist wearing shoes because what fun is that, and have food preferences. They are eager to kick and resist any changes or restrictions, which can be a little hard for first-time parents.

Know Who You Are

Not only do they learn to recognize you, but they also comprehend that you don't actually go away when you leave the room and will eventually come back. So they don't cry every time they see you leave the room. They also enjoy playing hide-and-seek and peek-a-boo as their problem-solving skills improve.

Recognize Themselves in the Mirror

This is another delightful milestone! Your baby finally recognizes the person they see in the mirror and enjoys the attention they get. To show how happy they are, they will try to be as interactive as possible with themselves in the mirror. They will smile and try to engage in conversation with it.

Visual

Vision is typically as sharp and clear as an adult's

Can watch objects that are moving fast

Shows sustained visual interest

Appears visually oriented at home— understanding where things are in his/her environment

Watches an object that he/she throws

Watches a ball when rolled back and forth with another

Sensory

Hearing is very accurate

Enjoys looking and listening at the same time (reading books, or listening to song while watching actions)

Loves exploring textures and engaging in messy play

Continues to explore things with hands and mouth, close visual inspection and manipulates objects to further investigate sights, sounds, textures.

Through exploration, baby continues to learn how to grade speed and pressure of movements such as lifting a cup to get to mouth smoothly.

Continues to develop food preferences, but enjoys a greater variety of smells and tastes— may take 10 tries before baby learns to like a new food.

Baby's vestibular system (located in the inner ear), vision, and the ability to process information about body position through muscles and joints and sense of touch continue to all coordinate together to help him orient in space, balance, and move efficiently to perform a task at hand.

Enjoys a wide variety of music/sounds, touch and movement play

Physical Development

The biggest milestone in terms of their motor skill development is that they will no longer require being held and will move on their own. Some kids start to walk even before they turn one, but there is nothing to worry about if they don't. They should be crawling, and that in itself is a remarkable thing to do. They will learn to push themselves using their elbows and knees and crawl for longer periods without getting drained out. What more can you expect?

Pull Themselves Up

Formerly, you might have had to pull them up to stand, but they are going to do so their own. They will hold onto some furniture pieces and pull themselves up. They will also learn to support their weight and enjoy staying up still for longer periods of time.

Pick Things Up from Below

Some kids are scared of the idea of bending and picking up things from the ground. If you recall correctly, they used to call upon you when something they wanted fell. Now, they will handle it on their own and bend to pick things up.

Sit for Much Longer

As their skeletal muscles become more flexible, they will be able to enjoy sitting for long periods and staying engaged in some activity. They will also be eager to use both their hands at once such as wanting to feed themselves or squishing things in between their fingers. They will enjoy playing with their food more than eating it.

Communication Skills

Your baby may not know all the right words, but they surely love to chat and do voice inflections. They will also be able to recognize your voice out of the many and look in the direction of where it is coming from. Other than that, they will be able to:

Pick Up New Words Fast

They will understand the meaning of many words such as nap, feed, food, play, yes, and no. They may also learn to nod or shake their heads to signal yes or no. Additionally, they will be less talkative now as they are becoming more specific with the choice of words they use and aim to learn the words that already exist rather than making up their own.

Enjoy Rhymes and Poems

Colors, shapes, and sounds have always fascinated them, but now that they can understand them better, they will enjoy them the most. They will try to mimic the steps or dance they see the characters on the screen doing or just make up their own to show how excited they are. They will also have favorites now that they are turning one. So parents should prepare themselves to hear one poem repeated a hundred times before they switch to the next one.

Communication Skills

Uses different hand movements or gestures to communicate wants and needs—pointing, reach to pick up, reach and hold hand toward desired object, bang or push at a toy to get repeated effect

Shakes head "no"

Signals or says "no" to unwanted or disliked food

May say a few single words other than "mama" or "dada"

Understands tone of voice has meanings

Understands several one step requests—"give me the ball", "look at the dog"

Says or tries to say the name of a food he/she wants

Understands "no-no" although may not comply

Jabbers long string of sounds with tone and inflection that sound like conversation

Intellectual Skills

Their ability to understand what object permanence is will improve. Their memory improves too, and they can find things hidden from them, unlike before.

Sensory Awareness

Most babies this age learn to feed themselves and prefer eating on their own. You can introduce some finger foods during this phase and let them eat them on their own. They have learned to grasp things between their thumb and fingers, so this should be easy for them.

Bang Blocks

Isn't that the most exciting thing for them to do? They love to bang the blocks and put their tiny hands into containers, drawers, and cabinets and take them out. They also love to poke at things to get a feel for the texture and shape.

Drink from a Cup

As they progress from taking the bottle to drinking from a cuppy or a cup, they will become more eager to take the latter. Of course, at first, they will require some assistance holding the cup in their hands, but they will soon become good at it.

Cooperates in Getting Dressed

Be it a diaper or dress change, they understand and accept the process when it happens, and their crying will eventually cease. When given the choice to choose their own clothes they will enjoy getting dressed and be cooperative too. They will happily extend their hands and feet to get out of the old clothes and into new ones.

Challenges This Month

- ***Spills and splashes:*** When you think about it, water really is a strange substance to explore. It can take on the shape of any container, but when poured out, it flattens instantly, forming a puddle that can shine back your reflection. It's no wonder babies delight in spilling liquid and splashing in it. Whenever you know your baby will be around a source of water, embrace the fun within reasonable limits and be ready with a change of clothing. (Never leave your baby unattended near water.)

•**Birthday party preparation:** Your baby will not understand the purpose of a birthday party celebrating his first year. Consider how comfortable he is around other people when you plan a party. If he gets nervous around large groups, a smaller, calmer party in a familiar location could be more baby-friendly.

When to Worry?

- Rarely shows excitement when looking at familiar faces
- Doesn't sit on its own
- Isn't interested in things and gets irritated fast
- Is still babbling and not saying any words
- Isn't motivated to walk with or without the support and prefers sitting or lying down

- Has poor hand-eye coordination

- Doesn't experience separation anxiety

Chapter 5: Montessori Baby From 0 To 12 Months

Before the birth

While in the womb a child dozes and awakens as indicated by his needs. He is brought into the world with the capacity to self-direct both dozing and eating and we can bolster this capacity by watching him cautiously. It is significant that he be benefited from interest instead of on a schedule (even though the interims will be near one another in the main days) and that the parents don't wake him when resting, or attempt to 'put' him to rest, releasing him to rest and wake up without anyone else. Steadily he will conform to the family plan. Whenever given a spot in a room and furthermore in the territories where the family goes through the day he will figure out how to put himself to rest and to wake up without anyone else, regardless of what is happening around him.

Sounds and songs

The child was glancing near, investigating the environment outwardly, and abruptly the music started to play. He kept as yet, looking toward the music, the CD player. Perceiving the intensity of the child's center, the mother sat similarly as still for quite a while, until the kid demonstrated her—by turning his head, moaning with fulfillment, and again concentrating on nature, that he had completed the process of tuning in to the music.

Kids ought to learn, as early in life as would be prudent, that music originates from a genuine human's activities; this present child's eyes move to and fro from the drummer foot and hand, the two wellsprings of sound. Parents should be singing each day (No one must be a Bonnie Raitt), and at whatever point conceivable give instrument to genuine instruments being played. This gives the child this present reality in the entirety of its melodic potential outcomes and gives a model to his future. This is significant work. Age 5 months.

Toys to suck and grab

When the child can sit up the hands are liberated for significant work and we ought to accommodate this need. Over numerous long stretches of the Montessori Assistants to
Infancy work far and wide materials, made of normal items rather than plastic, have been built up that appeal the kid and simultaneously give an intention to focus, critical thinking, and the redundancy of developments of the hand and arm and entire body that help the mental and physical improvement of the kid.

Sign Language

Babies will feel a desire to communicate long before their lips and tongues are strong enough to do so. I find that many parents who are resistant to sign language fear that it may be too complex. The secret to baby signing is to teach 8 basic words, incorporating them one at a time: 1. Drink 2. More

3. Need to eliminate

4. Finished

5. Hungry

6. Toy

7. Mom

8. Dad

Studies demonstrate that babies who learn basic sign language at about six months develop more cognitive passageways sooner, have higher I.Q's, and may have fewer tantrums. Maria Montessori believed that anything that empowers your baby to communicate their needs and feelings is a valuable resource.

Yes Environment Instead of a No Environment

During their maturity, babies have a tendency to find just about everything in their environment appealing. Arrange your living room, kitchen, bathroom, hallways, and bedrooms in both an *accommodating* and *aesthetically pleasing* manner. Start with a single room. Could a crawling baby explore without your interruption? If not, consider making some simple changes. For instance: If there are bookshelves that baby could reach up and pull books off of, consider relocating the books to higher shelves and\or storage. If there is a priceless heirloom on the coffee table, why not relocate it to the mantle?

Arrange each room so that there is no need to redirect.

A *Yes Environment* will ward off problems before they start, and will ease the mind of the parents when baby is exploring her new world. Positive reinforcement is always favored to discipline.

Music

Play music for your baby at set times, keep volume low and bear in mind that babies developing ears are more sensitive to sound than adults. When experiencing music, many newborns may not seem to respond for the first few months, but have patience. W.A. Mozart and J.S. Bach are the most studied composers, and their works seem to have consistent positive results. Others composers who have gained acclaim are F. Chopin, L.V. Beethoven, and J. Brahms. For best results, compile a list -one track at a time, for one week. Introducing a single piece (as opposed to an entire album or an endless stream) will allow your baby to make associations faster than simply playing a wide spectrum of pieces every day.

Exposure to certain classical music improves spatial reasoning, helps form neural pathways, calms baby, and stimulates the immune system. As a pianist, baby lover, and classical music fanatic, I have included my recommended playlist. Feel free to deviate from it according to your own taste.

Activity: Pouring Objects

Although often not seen as toys, pouring can be a supreme pleasure for infants. Begin by allowing your infant to pour solid objects such as buttons, nuts, or uncooked beans between two bowls. Once finished, allow him to dive his hands into the bowls and squish the contents. Then when you feel he is ready, graduate to pouring water.

Pouring lengthens attention span, facilitates cause and effect, promotes cognitive skills, improves depth perception, and familiarizes infants with the concept of ratios.

Communication

Except for when your baby is sleeping, waking, nursing, or upset, you should speak to him in a clear, direct, and warm voice. Resist the urge to talk at your baby, instead, communicate with him. Ask him questions and observe his responses. You may be surprised by the nonverbal answers you'll get to the questions you ask with sincerity. Practice repeating phrases 7-10 times per day; use the same sentences and the same tone of voice. Obvious choices might be. "Hello my sweet (babies name) I am (your name) and I love you very much." Another exercise would be to practice using the same phrase at specific times of the day: "Good morning (babies name) did you enjoy your breakfast this morning?"
Speaking to your baby in a similar manner (for the first few months) will help their cognition and speech recognition.

First books

Intentional discussions about their day, their surroundings are vital. Books can build up a propensity for conversing with the kid and utilize an assortment of words and articulations. We cherish books with surfaces in them for little fingers to play with. Eric Carle's books have exceptionally appealing illustrations and are interactive.

Looking in a mirror

At the point when an adult holds a kid's hand to walk the child winds up reliant on the adult for practice that he can do whenever if a bar like this one is given. Also, the hidden message can be "I need you to stroll." rather than "Your phase of advancement is ideal for you. You are fine only the manner in which you are." it is greatly improved to give an environment in which a kid can choose when and for to what extent to rehearse each new skill, for example, pulling up.

Be a Model to your Child

As your child matures, she will begin to take after you. If you speak impolitely to her, if you curse at people in traffic, if you argue in a petty manner with your spouse, she will absorb how you are behaving, and, if your bad behavior is consistent, she will begin to display the same attributes, albeit on a smaller scale. On the other hand, if you are patient, courteous, kind, tender, and loving, your child is more likely to display those qualities.

If you devote yourself to being a better parent, your child will help you become one.

Your House is a Museum

At about 3 months, make it a weekly practice to take your baby on a tour of your house. Act as if you were a museum guide giving a tour, pausing at places of interest. Allow your baby a moment to take in what is before them. Then, briefly explain what you are showing them. Dedicate extra time to areas that baby displays interest in. If there is something that you are fond of, share it with your baby. Do you have a sculpture or a stained glass window in your house? How about a fountain in your yard? If not, don't fret; your newborn will be equally enthralled by the sink in your kitchen and the pine tree in your front yard.

This practice facilitates the sensory stimulation that is so important to baby's growth and development.

Movement, from crawling to coordination

For a considerable length of time, a child has been investigating the environment outwardly and can barely wait to taste and touch! The drive to push ahead in any capacity conceivable additionally assembles a solid mind; "creeping" and crawling get ready for reading and composing and thinking. The best thing we can offer the child at this safe is a protected and fascinating condition and opportunity to move without being hurried or intruded. This is significant work. (4-5 months)
NOTE: Some individuals invert the terms "crawling" and "creeping."

Children everywhere throughout the world display similar phases of advancement when they have a domain that supports them. A sleeping cushion on the floor, opportunity to move and investigate in an exceptionally protected spot. This little Polish child demonstrates to us the entire body shaking stage that goes before crawling, the equalization and certainty to build up the capacities to get off of his floor bed, and no uncertainty the energy to move from the room to the more extensive universe of the home.

Language and first words

At the point when a mother or father addresses a youngster merciful, with the right language and in a typical manner of speaking (not utilizing infant talk), and clarifies what she/he is doing (for this situation securing a sweater) the kid naturally realizes he is being regarded a completely cognizant individual.

small objects

In the primary days and long stretches of life, the kid is seriously keen on watching and looking. From the outset, his capacity to the center is the separation between his eyes and the mother's face during nursing. Before long he is keen on watching mobiles that move delicately in the breeze. Mobiles ought to have close to 5 objects and they ought to be genuine, for example, butterflies, feathered creatures, or fish—things that travel through the air or water. (2.5 months).

Social life

Maria Montessori saw that all children learn according to natural, worked in phases of advancement. Children under six years of age are building up a personality, or feeling of self.

They will regularly like to work separately. They may work by other children, they may even watch and gain from other children, yet they are best ready to concentrate and learn without anyone else. As the child gets more established, they grow a develop more of an interest in adapting cooperatively. The Montessori Method regards these common tendencies of the developing kid. Children have the opportunity to work independently from anyone else when they have to. In like manner, children can work in gatherings and help each other.

Evaluate What's Working

The Montessori method is a framework for developing a healthy, autonomous, wellrounded child. Because every baby is unique it is recommended that you evaluate what is (and what is not) working with your individual baby every three months, and then adapt or modify any of the bullet points above. The Montessori System should not be taken as Gospel; it should be regarded as a method that is constantly evolving, just like babies are.

Evaluating what's working, and modifying practices and environments accordingly will help ensure that your baby grows up to be as happy, healthy, strong, as they can be.

Conclusion

Thank you for reading this book. The aspiration of every parent is to train children that are
disciplined and virtuous. Every parent you are ever likely to meet will want their children to grow up to be good ambassadors of the family, to represent a value-based upbringing, and bring joy and personal fulfilment both to themselves and to the parents.

Babies are trying to let us, and in particular their parents, know that they have specific physical and emotional needs, and that if we can only begin to understand what it is they are trying to tell us, we will be in a much better position to help them and ourselves.

It is normal to feel scared while also feeling excited to become a new parent. Both feelings are incredibly justified. Once you get into the swing of things, though, you will be able to build up your confidence and take every little smile and giggle as a sign that you are doing something right!

And that is what this text provides. It is written with both parents and children in mind. Great effort has been made to fill the pages with the adequate knowledge you need in the parenting of your toddlers, and to make it accessible in language and organization. It enables the deepest connection between parents and their toddlers on the one hand, and a virtuous growth of the children on the other hand. This study guide was created to help parents become duly equipped in the training of your infant. It is purely and exclusively educational, and it will be wrong to use the content of this study guide to diagnose health or psychological problems.

Good luck.